SPORTS FOR LIFE

SPORTS FOR LIFE

Fitness Training,
Nutrition, and
Injury Prevention

Robert Buxbaum, M.D.
Lyle J. Micheli, M.D.

with illustrations by Jeremy Elkin

BEACON PRESS Boston

Grateful acknowledgment is made to the following: Lenore R. Zohman, M.D., for permission to reprint the chart "Maximal Attainable Heart Rate and Target Zone" that appears in the brochure *Beyond Diet: Exercise Your Way to Fitness and Heart Health*, Lenore R. Zohman, M.D., CPC International Inc., Englewood Cliffs, N.J.; and The Mountaineers for permission to reprint their "Wind Chill Chart" from *Medicine for Mountaineering*, edited by James A. Wilkerson, M.D., Seattle, WA, 1975.

Beacon Press books are published under the auspices of the Unitarian Universalist Association

Published simultaneously in Canada by Fitzhenry & Whiteside Limited, Toronto

Printed in the United States of America

(hardcover) 9 8 7 6 5 4 3 2 1
(paperback) 9 8 7 6 5 4 3 2

Library of Congress Cataloging in Publication Data

Buxbaum, Robert, 1930-
Sports for life.
Bibliography: p.
Includes index.
1. Sports. 2. Physical fitness. I. Micheli, Lyle J., 1940- joint author. II. Title. GV706.8.B89 1979 613.7
79-51150
ISBN 0-8070-2162-8
ISBN 0-8070-2163-6 pbk.

Preface

AS PHYSICIANS with a commitment to exercise, one of us a sports medicine specialist, the other an internist with a general population of patients, we have a unique opportunity to view the role of fitness in society. We must also admit that our perceptions as observant human beings are not unbiased. Our own personal interest in the field leads us to want change to occur, when in fact the change may come more slowly than we hope.

But general interest in fitness and life sports is definitely growing—growing in unexpected ways. It is to those who wish to become more active, to combat the ill effects of our highly mechanized society, to avoid injuries on the road to health that we address this book. We hope you can use it as a medical sports adviser and a training coach.

Robert Buxbaum, M.D.
Lyle J. Micheli, M.D.

Contents

SPORTS FOR LIFE

I
BODY BASICS

Americans have begun to move down the path to increasing their physical capacities. They are no longer content to be told to stop a sport when something hurts. Doctors who advise their patients to "put away their shoes" are not likely to be consulted again. Instead, people are looking for help in maintaining programs that avoid injury and that treat injuries when they occur so that the participant does not have to give up or postpone the sport. Knowledge of the basic elements of our bodies in motion is essential in reaching these goals. A sensitivity to the need for muscle and tendon conditioning is essential to help lower the chances of injury and disability due to sports-related events.

The purpose of this book is to explain, in simple terms, what happens when the body moves. This is not a textbook on physiology but a guide that provides basic information to help you reach your own personal fitness goals and enhance the use and enjoyment of your body.

1. Lifetime Fitness and Sports

THE SURGE OF INTEREST in fitness and lifetime sports has passed beyond the point at which it might be considered a fad. The growing number of participants is testimony to our apparently deep-seated need to experience motion—not that linked to the machine, but the body's own. Rediscovering how the body works has brought a new sense of control and pleasure to millions of people.

This understanding has come about without a lot of medical input. The fitness movement has been a campaign of the people, not of the physicians. Only recently has the medical profession begun to adjust to this trend; it is our perception that we doctors still have a long way to go before we completely understand what motivates people to become fit, how the body functions during physical stress, to what limits of performance the body can be pushed, what the benefits of fitness are, and how to prevent those untoward events that occur from overexercising and those injuries that result from participating in sports. With the millions joining the fitness movement, these are important issues to confront, and there are simply not enough qualified medical professionals available to advise on them.

We believe that a well-informed public is the best safeguard against exercise misuse, as well as the proper base for the development of national programs to improve the fitness of the country. Furthermore, an understanding of one's body in motion and the role of training, conditioning, and injury prevention will help shift the burden of health promotion from the medical profession to the consumer, where it belongs. There are times when a doctor is needed, but more often it is the runner, swimmer, or cyclist himself/herself who knows more about the subject than the medical professional.

All physical activity starts with a nerve impulse from the brain. Motivation and intellect are thus intimately linked with the movement process, since without them no activity can take place. Even though the rhythmic movements of sports are repetitive and may seem to be automatic, they are affected by training, environment, the ability to adjust to differing circumstances, and—as we will emphasize—physical endurance.

This aspect of physical activity—endurance—is just beginning to yield to scientific investigation. It holds the promise of being one of the most important subjects of study in the latter part of this century. How it affects the health of people, how it may help to change poor health habits into healthy behavior, and what it can do to affect the psyche are all valid subjects for investigation and development. This research is in its infancy; the present enthusiastic claims for fitness must yield eventually to a rational scientific appraisal.

As physicians who believe that fitness is vital for good health, we have an admitted bias in favor of human movement. In our professional capacities we regularly observe injuries related to sports and see people before they begin fitness programs as well as those already participating in them. We are impressed with the kind of determination people bring to the physician's office now compared to the lack of interest we saw just a few years ago. Runners want to run *through* the pain of injury, middle-aged people want to know if it is safe to begin exercising, patients announce—proudly—that they have begun walking, skiing, running, swimming, playing racquet sports, or jumping rope for their health. No longer can a physician tell a patient to stop exercising because it is not appropriate at his/her age; the patient will find a physician who will help and support the patient rather than one who will suggest sedentary alternatives.

We see changes in the pattern of injury too. The various

sprains, strains, and overuse syndromes that have always been the athlete's lot are now much more a part of everyone's daily life. What was once locker-room shop talk about knee, foot or muscle problems now appears in conversation among dedicated amateurs, almost anywhere, any time.

It is to this kind of participant that *Sports for Life* is addressed. We will show that it is not only good to exercise, but that it is also possible to construct a varied and interesting program that can be changed from season to season. We will also show the amateur athlete how to regulate the right amount of demand upon the heart and lungs so as to foster good health. With a variety of appropriate choices, the participant need not become immobilized. The runner hobbled with Achilles' tendinitis and the saddle-weary cyclist can turn to other activities to keep their hearts strong.

It has become increasingly clear that along with all the other hazards of daily life, physical *inactivity* ranks high. Until recently lack of historical perspective has led many of us to assume that a life-style depending on machines and processed foods is immutable and somehow good—a mark of progress. But we are now beginning to see that in the past several generations alarming changes have taken place in the nature and incidence of disease and disability as a result of the cultural characteristics of the Machine Age. Heart disease, once an insignificant statistic on the disease horizon, is now the principal cause of death for Americans. We know that this disease and others are associated with the way we live. Casting aside a sedentary life-style can lead to a lowered risk of premature death and disability.

We all have a stake in seeing that changes take place. The economics of the medical marketplace are forcing us to find alternatives to those extremely expensive late-stage attempts at diagnosis and cure that doctors currently employ. Some governments, facing spiraling medical care costs, have sought to put a lid on spending. Others have looked to health promotion. In many instances, it has become clear that physical fitness has a central role to play, both as a primary method of disease prevention and as a way of motivating people toward an all-around healthier way of living.

It is our belief that Americans want and deserve a true *fitness policy*, that is, a concerted effort on the part of government, health and recreation agencies, schools, and employers that fosters the individual's efforts to fulfill his/her potential for lifetime physical fitness. This effort should not be limited by a person's level of skill or intellect; physical handicaps should be a reason to encourage fitness, not discourage it.

It is our feeling that we are not witnessing a short-lived physical fitness phenomenon but rather the expression of a deeply rooted need for the body to move, to break free of such restraints as the automobile and spectator sports that have enslaved us. The purpose of this book is to open the door for those interested in physical movement so they may understand and experience the pleasure that comes with activity, to help them know how to prepare for it as well as how to guard against the problems that can arise in its pursuit.

Central to our approach is the notion that movement and its effects are pleasurable. While there is a need for some technical background for each sport described, the essential quality in the pursuit of fitness should be *joy*. If that is forgotten in a grim search for fitness, the essential justification for movement will be lost. We hope that in the current search for fitness, the reader will remember that the major sustaining force comes from within each individual.

People engage in sports for a variety of reasons: company, the prestige and sense of accomplishment provided, the feeling of change and muscular development. Perhaps the most compelling reason to become fit is to develop a sense of control over one's own body. In an era in which so many events are out of any one person's control or even understanding, it is important to be able to shape and influence the workings of as complex an organism as one's body, even in a limited way. This is particularly important when the shaping is in the direction of better health, in contrast, say, to that which occurs under the effect of alcohol or drugs.

We have written this book in part because we believe that, if our sedentary life-style has led to a huge increase in inactivity-related diseases, the logical mode of prevention is *activity*. It is that simple. The millions of dollars of lost productivity due to low back pain, for example, would cease to be so large a problem if we paid attention to strengthening the back from an early age onward. As it happens, most of the current effort is spent in trying to correct the problem once it has made its appearance, after years of neglect. In regard to heart disease, there are now over thirty years of studies clearly linking physical activity with a lessening of the incidence and death rate for the disorder. Even leisure-time exercise carried out on a modest scale seems to have a protective effect. Whatever one might say about statistics—they can show only *association*, not cause and effect—they clearly strengthen the belief that fitness is important, perhaps preeminent, in heart disease prevention.

Just as important is the weight of evidence from the laboratory. Studies of the heart, made while the body is in motion, show that the well-trained heart is a much more efficient organ than one that has not been so trained. Training is a very specific process, and underlies every activity described in this book. Apart from heart disease prevention, training helps the heart work smoothly and without undue risk when emergencies or stress occur. This is as vital for the person whose job requires him/her to be in a position of stress as it is for the individual who wishes to run or swim. It is similarly important for anyone who simply wants to get up out of a chair to take a brisk walk or climb stairs. It has been claimed that by the 1950s the average American male could not climb a flight of stairs without becoming breathless. Perhaps there has been a reversal of that trend, but as a nation we still worry more about high performance in automobiles than in people.

The body is unique in that the more it is stressed—up to a point—the better it functions. Its parts do not wear out in the same fashion as machines'. Stress placed on muscles, including the heart, tends to make them work more efficiently during nonstressful times. The *neglect* of muscles, on the other hand, causes them to become weak and soft. Bones depend upon constant stress to maintain their structural integrity. Joints are better lubricated and have a wider range of motion if they are kept in motion.

FITNESS FOR WHAT?

For everyone who is interested in fitness, there are attainable goals. Ultimately, the only useful competition is with oneself. Measurement of that performance can be satisfying and self-sustaining. Understanding the elements of performance can add further gratification.

While cardiovascular (heart and breathing) endurance is a common thread in training, it is important to understand that training for a given sport does not automatically confer fitness for another. Running, for instance, is not training for jumping rope or swimming, though it may contribute somewhat to a higher level of heart conditioning for these sports. Similarly, injuries that occur in one sport are not always to be found in another.

The changes that take place with sports can be revelatory. Cardiovascular improvement (to be described in detail later) consists of a lowered heart rate, more efficient pumping of the heart muscle, greater tolerance for stress, and a feeling of heightened energy and capacity for work. Hand in hand go an increased sense of physical confidence, better sleep, improved digestion, and, some say, a better sex life. Finally, there is the intriguing possibility of better mental health. Fragmentary but important new information suggests that anxiety and depression are lessened through regular exercise and that the "natural high" of which many people speak may have its basis in some hormonal change that takes place as a result of fitness activities.

As we have stated, the secrets of the body in motion are just beginning to emerge. How different from the study of the body at rest, which was the physiology taught generations of medical students, and how important, since the body is constructed for motion, that the marvelous and complex interrelationship of heart, lungs, blood, muscle, and skeleton, with all the supporting and buffering organs, was meant to comprise an organism in more or less constant motion.

Our message is aimed at men and women who wish to

start a personal fitness program through sports or to improve on one already in progress. It is designed to help minimize the risk of injury. We do not try, except for a few comments, to deal with the immense and important area of school sports and physical education; that could be the subject of another book, or series of books. Our hope is that women and men can find new ways to improve their bodies through physical fitness and that by setting such an example their children will wish to participate too.

GETTING GOING

Perhaps the weakest strand of our knowledge about fitness is that concerned with what makes people want to run, swim, or otherwise extend their physical capacities. Our record of success in getting people to stop smoking is poor, and weight-reduction programs, if they are honest about reporting their statistics, must admit huge failure rates. So there is little in the scientific world that can tell us how to encourage people to stay in a lifetime fitness program. Nonetheless, it is worth the effort involved, for both economic and health reasons. Furthermore, the management of fitness programs may require vastly different skills from those necessary to run successful antismoking and diet programs. Fitness is a positive goal, a "taking on" rather than a "giving up."

While there is evidence that fitness is a useful (and nonpharmaceutical) method of treating anxiety and depression, current studies leave much to be desired and should not be overinterpreted. Here, as in all aspects of fitness, one must be wary of unsupported or overblown claims. Runners who compare their sport to a massive religious experience lack perspective, particularly if their most recent revelation prior to running was in an automobile. Fitness, it can be stated, will probably assist people in feeling better, at least at certain times, and it is probably true that, if training lapses, the participant will feel less well until he/she resumes it. Beyond that, it is hard at this point to make many firm assertions about mental benefits.

There is also a role for fitness promotion. Perhaps some sort of mass advertising that would make fitness attractive to people while teaching them about it should be initiated. An emphasis upon Olympian performance is not productive; a campaign addressed to ordinary people with less exalted goals would be best.

There is a need for groups to function in this area as well; beginning exercisers need the encouragement and reinforcement that groups provide. Talking about feelings with regard to fitness is as important as the activity itself. Fitness should be a social activity in any case, and the firm date made with a friend to run is the best insurance against the tendency to drop out.

For some participants, there will come a time when the process is so internalized that no outside stimulus is needed. An internal clock will announce that it is time to dive into a pool, go out for a jog, or practice jumping rope. At that point, the learning process is complete, and the body's chemistry and physiology are on their own.

For that fit individual, equipped with a good working knowledge of the body, informed about nutrition, aware of the hazards of physical movement and of the body's limits, the process of becoming fit has achieved one of its highest goals; the development of a smoothly functioning organism developed to its highest physical potential.

Until a person has reached that state, he/she may need a lot of encouragement. This might be pressure from friends, family, or colleagues who are themselves active. Physicians' advice has been shown to be extremely important. But the capacity to stay with the program is a product of many factors, including the setting of new goals, different for each individual. Above all as a motivating force is the sense of *enjoyment.*

In some countries, it is difficult to escape the barrage of propaganda aimed at overcoming unfitness; the TRIM movement in Europe, for example, tends to use billboards and television advertising as principal ways of changing people's minds. The average Swede knows that it is healthy to bike to work; in addition, facilities there are so well developed that no one lives or works more than a short distance from superb indoor and outdoor fitness programs. Canadians have been exposed to a highly sophisticated television advertising campaign aimed at getting everyone to move, and the Health and Welfare Ministry has distributed thousands of copies of the Canadian Fit-Kit, an imaginative package that includes a fitness self-assessment, a record, and materials written by Professor Per-Olof Åstrand that are readable and practical.

Åstrand is widely regarded in medical and physiologic circles as the most articulate spokesperson for the advancement of fitness. Chairman of the Department of Physiology at the Karolinska Institute in Stockholm, he has had an immense impact upon the growth of exercise physiology and its application to public policy in his homeland as well as elsewhere around the world. In a sense, this book would have been impossible without his contribution.

Åstrand believes that, based upon his and others' laboratory investigations, the human body can be brought to a state of highly improved physical fitness through a relatively modest investment of time and energy. His studies of top athletes and others provide the necessary scientific basis for the assertion that a thirty-minute, three-day-a-week investment can serve as the basis for significantly improved cardiovascular performance.

Self-rewards for performance can play a very important part in keeping up a program; some people give themselves "points." A diary can be helpful. Whatever the system used, whether it is gold stars, special recognition, or T-shirts, it should encourage people to feel that they are not as much themselves when they don't exercise regularly.

WOMEN'S PARTICIPATION

Fortunately for the fitness of over 50 percent of our population, the historic sexual imbalance in physical activity is changing rapidly. More and more women are finding a new and lasting interest and enjoyment in recreational sports. While it is true—because many women are new to the field—that their rate of injury has been higher than that of males, this should begin equalizing, particularly after women have shed the cultural inhibitions that have held them back for so long. From our experience as sports medicine physicians we believe that the only reason for women's higher injury rate is that many are "new" athletes, lacking expertise in both basic physical training techniques as well as specific sports skills. Today, women participate not only in those sports that have been considered traditionally for females—field hockey, softball, basketball, and gymnastics, for example—but they are also entering those previously considered for males only. These "new female sports" include soccer, ice hockey, baseball, rugby, and even gridiron football. The woman jogger and cyclist has joined the male as a common sight on city streets.

There are a number of important social forces underlying this increased participation. Equal rights legislation, such as Title IX of the Education Amendments of 1972, and specific state legislation require that males and females be provided equal access to educational facilities, including gymnasiums and playing fields, as well as access to instruction. This is true at all levels of schooling, from primary school through college. In 1975, more than 1.3 million high school girls participated in twenty-seven interscholastic sports, a 59 percent increase from 1973.

Female candidates participate in the rigorous physical and athletic activities of the military academies, and women compete for athletic scholarships at universities. Feminists have emphasized the value of recognition and the resulting enhancement of self-esteem that arise from athletic participation and achievement, heretofore a totally male domain. Finally, weight-reduction programs, most of them aimed at women (although equally applicable to males), have begun to place more emphasis on exercise, and cosmetic and beauty firms have begun to stress the athletic, healthy look. As a result of these various trends, exercise and sports participation for women have become accepted and even fashionable.

Whatever the motivation, the appearance of great numbers of new women athletes has caused questions to be raised regarding appropriate techniques for fitness and training for the female athlete. While some have questioned the ability of women to participate in progressive training activities, the evidence, by and large, continues to support the conclusion that women can safely follow exactly the same guidelines for fitness training as men—namely, specificity, overload and rest, and slow progressive training.

We have been asked, are there different cardiovascular endurance standards for men and women? Until quite recently, it was assumed that the female lacked the endurance of the male. Individual feats, such as Gertrude Ederle's setting of the English Channel swimming record in 1926, were felt to be bizarre and atypical. Even today, Olympic track competition does not permit women's events in excess of two kilometers. Kathy Switzer, the first woman to run in the Boston Marathon, was able to do so in 1967 only by successfully evading Marathon officials who attempted to physically restrain her at the outset of the race. The anecdotal evidence often precedes the laboratory confirmation; athletic performance has frequently illuminated physiologic principles that only later become confirmed through research and investigation. The more than five hundred women who have completed the grueling Boston Marathon offer the most convincing evidence that women, with proper training and conditioning, can safely endure this level of cardiovascular stress, and the success of highly trained female mountaineering teams in the Himalayas and elsewhere has laid to rest the myth of female weakness.

Indeed, laboratory evidence now firmly supports the theory that the physiologic response of highly trained women to endurance stress is very similar to that of their male counterparts and far exceeds that of the untrained and unfit male in our society. Further diminishing the traditional but overstated superiority of males, it has been suggested by some that women, who possess a higher percentage of body weight in the form of fat than men, may have an enhanced ability to metabolize this body fat and use it for energy. Thus, after the usual two and a half to three hours of endurance stress which is known to use up most males' stores of both liver and muscle glycogen, as well as sugars, the female may still be utilizing energy from her fat tissues. While recent investigations show that *both* the highly trained male and female have an enhanced ability to use storage fat as fuel, such research only serves to suggest that sex, per se, has little to do with the capability for high endurance training.

The well-known difference in muscular strength between men and women has often been used as a justification for excluding women from certain sports, particularly those involving contact, as it is assumed that the physically weaker female would be at a higher risk of injury than her male teammate or opponent.

It has been well established that muscle bulk or size is associated with higher levels of male hormones, and weightlifters and body-builders have often used the muscle-building properties of supplemental male hormones (a practice that deserves condemnation). It has not been demonstrated, however, that muscle *strength* increases directly proportional to muscle *bulk*. While muscle strength and size increase in the young male at puberty, this effect may be due to more than just the rising level of male hormones at that stage of development. The lack of increase of muscle development in pubertal women, which is well demonstrated in this culture, has been attributed in the past to hormonal influences. It is noteworthy, however, that in the past the observed differences in upper body strength between males and females have been much more pronounced than the differences in average lower body strength. In addition, despite a relatively lower average of muscle strength (again more pronounced in the upper body), the female, when exposed to systematic weight training, shows a pattern of strength development very similar to that of comparably trained males.

The often dramatic improvement in athletic performance and lower rate of injury resulting from weight-training programs for women have been well documented by research. These studies, moreover, show that this gain in muscle strength is not accompanied by a disproportionate increase in muscle bulk in women, an important cosmetic issue for many participants. While it remains to be seen whether the upper limits of attainable muscle strength of women will match those of men, it is evident that women are not nearly at as much of a disadvantage as once thought insofar as their ability to increase their strength with weight training is concerned.

Part of the explanation for the difference in male and female strength may derive from social, rather than physical, factors. Studies of young children show no significant differences in motor behavior between girls and boys, particularly with regard to strength, reflexes, and endurance. But in the past, our society has dictated significantly different pathways of development and roles for males and females after puberty. The male—particularly the athletic male—has been encouraged to develop his upper extremities with much more muscle work and training than the female. Children who actively climb trees or playground equipment together at age nine thereafter tend to follow different, sex-dictated paths. At thirteen it has been felt quite appropriate for males to lift weights, while females watch admiringly. On the other hand, there has been less differentiation in roles as they affect the lower extremities. A young woman, while learning to behave "like a lady," might have abandoned tree climbing or throwing a ball, but not standing, walking, or running. This may help to explain why such small differences in the lower body strength exist between the sexes.

It can be safely concluded, then, that both the cardiovascular and musculoskeletal training of women involved in athletics can be very similar to that of men. At the same time, the need for proper flexibility exercises must be emphasized. While there is some evidence that women are, on the whole, more flexible than men, there is no question that such culturally determined activities as wearing shoes with high heels tend to affect flexibility, in this case by making the heel cords and calf muscles of women relatively tighter. Thus, for the female athlete, heel cord stretching and flexibility exercises in particular are recommended for most sport activities in order to improve technique and prevent injury.

FEMALE INJURIES AND THEIR PREVENTION

It can be seen that similar types of injuries occur in men and women, although the frequency of some types varies according to sex as well as in specific cause. Sex-specific problems are few in number, however. Breast injuries, long thought to bar women from participating in contact sports, are probably among the rarest injuries seen in women's athletics. A survey of college sports revealed several reports of breast bruises but no serious injuries. In the experience of the Children's Hospital Medical Center Sports Medicine Division in Boston, which followed four women's rugby clubs for a period of three years, not one significant breast injury occurred. Nevertheless, breast protection continues to be a concern, and occasionally a rule change such as allowing women soccer players to protect their chests from a kicked ball with crossed arms will occur. And certain women's hockey leagues use special chest protectors. On the whole, however, there seems to be little need for concern in this regard.

In the area of breast *support*, special athletic bras have been marketed in the hope of minimizing discomfort rather than providing protection. However, a survey of women marathon runners has shown that as many say they are comfortable without support as say they feel support is useful. This could be a result, of course, of breast size alone.

With respect to the genitalia, female reproductive organs have a much greater degree of natural protection from athletic injury than those of males, and serious sports-related injuries to the female sexual organs are extremely rare.

Menstruation appears to be no significant barrier to women's participation or performance in sports, and some studies have shown that vigorous athletic participation has caused a decrease in menstrual complaints. Certain highly trained female athletes who participate in endurance sports have noted menstrual irregularity as a result of intensive training, but have not noted any permanent impairment of reproductive or sexual function. Specifically, the disappearance of menstruation has been known to occur in some highly conditioned female athletes from training alone. Training should not, of course, be assumed to be the only possible cause, and a medical examination to rule out pituitary dysfunction or other causes is in order.

There is no question that we can and do see many of the same types of musculoskeletal (muscle and bone) injuries in women as in men—including fractures, dislocations, and contusions. These injuries, usually the result of major trauma, have a similar cause in both sexes and are managed identically.

Another group of injuries, however, exist. These are the result of recurrent microtrauma, such as the constant impact of footfall in running, particularly on pavement, or the repetitive throwing of a ball or hitting a ball with a racquet. Overuse syndromes are increasingly a problem for the woman athlete, and include stress fractures, problems of the kneecap, certain tendinitis and bursitis problems, "tennis elbow," and the elusive, mysterious, but painful "shin splint."

An overuse syndrome is usually the result of the interaction of several factors: an error in training, such as proceeding with too much intensity, too rapidly; an anatomic malalignment of the bones or joints, as in the instance of a previous injury badly healed; imbalance of the tendons of the arm or leg, either in flexibility or strength; inadequate equipment, such as poorly fitted or designed running shoes; or the use of improper surface, such as concrete rather than asphalt or dirt.

The newer woman athlete's susceptibility to these problems seems to occur because of a lack of long-term preparation for vigorous sports training. It takes years to condition the bones and soft tissues of the extremities—male or female—for vigorous athletic activities. For example, classic ballet, with its rich and ancient tradition of physical training techniques, requires three or more years of progressive training before a student is allowed advanced technique, including *en pointe*.

In the past, the relatively low levels of athletic training

and participation available for women in our society rendered them significantly less fit than men, both in cardiovascular (heart/lung) and musculoskeletal functions. While it takes only a few months, at most, for the heart and lungs to achieve higher levels of fitness, muscles and bones, and in particular the bones of the extremities, take much longer to remodel and strengthen themselves in response to physical demands. As a result, a higher rate of injury is seen in recreational women athletes than in men at the present time. Given the historic basis of these differences, however, it is likely that they will progressively disappear, as athletic fitness and training for children and young adults begins to cast aside traditional sexual stereotypes and to treat men and women with more evenhandedness.

A good example of this principle in action exists in downhill skiing. Early studies of injuries showed that the novice woman skier sustained two or three times the rate of injury compared to the male novice. However, more recent studies indicate that this difference has been wiped out. Obviously, the difference could not have been due to hormones, inherent muscle strength, or anything else having to do with an immutable distinction between the sexes.

In summary, then, there are no basic differences in the cardiovascular, musculoskeletal, or flexibility characteristics in women and men that affect their preparation for recreational sport activities. Since, however, the individual woman may have had a less intense exposure to previous musculoskeletal stress and training, she may have to proceed at a slower and more deliberate rate of training initially. She can, however, expect to obtain equivalent levels of fitness, training, and enjoyment if she follows proper training techniques.

Our approach, then, is to encourage the fullest and widest participation by *people*—male or female—in the challenge of lifetime fitness activities. Many will turn to sports, in the traditional sense; many others will be drawn to individual activities whose only challenge is the drive to do better, or whose major justification is the sense of fulfillment and increased energy felt through regular participation. In addition, we feel that everyone should have enough basic information to allow him/her to know how to become well conditioned for an activity, and to prevent injuries. But most of all we want to encourage the largest number of people possible to take advantage of the activity potential—often latent and poorly used—in their bodies. We hope that *Sports for Life* will help to bring this about.

2. Training Your Heart

CALORIES ARE HIGH in the consciousness of many people, and almost everyone is familiar with the term. The calorie (actually, *kilo*calorie) is a word derived from thermodynamics and is used to represent the amount of heat needed to warm up a specified amount of water. It is a useful, shorthand way of talking about the energy food contains, and can also apply to energy expenditure.

Since energy output relates directly to body weight, heavier people burn more calories (and therefore use more oxygen in the process) for a given type of exertion than thin people. For whatever satisfaction it may afford, a fat person walking a mile will burn off more calories than his/her thinner counterpart doing the same amount of exercise.

The energy we get from food is stored in muscle tissues—whether the heart or skeletal muscles—and is used to power muscular contraction. Triggered by nerve impulses, ATP (a highly charged source of energy in the muscle cell) is released, and the molecular structure of the muscle fiber, arranged like the familiar metal spring, contracts, pulling the attached bone into its new position; alternately, the cells relax, allowing the bone to return to its previous arrangement (or to be pulled in a new direction by a set of opposing muscles).

The heart is a somewhat special case; it isn't attached to bone, and since it must pump constantly, it is only partially under the influence of the brain and reflexes, which can modify but not interfere with its primary pumping action (unless disease of the brain occurs, and even then the heart is likely to manage perfectly well). The heart can do this because it has its own internal electrical system, which fires impulses at regular intervals, setting off the complex pump, with its valves and chambers, and thereby sending oxygen-rich blood to the entire body. Although it is self-stimulated, the heart is subject to some variations in rate and rhythm by chemicals, psychological factors, and training.

When energy output occurs, the heart is the organ ultimately responsible for our ability to carry out the tasks required. An output of several thousand calories requires a strong and well-functioning heart; the strain upon the heart itself depends on whether the demand occurs over a long or short period, whether it involves a few or many muscles, and whether or not there are any other organs actively competing for the oxygen being delivered. The method of energy metabolism that uses oxygen delivered by the action of the heart is called *aerobic metabolism.*

AEROBIC AND ANAEROBIC METABOLISM

Skeletal muscles are able to function both with and without oxygen—the only organs of the body capable of so doing. (However, their most efficient mode of function is aerobic—with oxygen.) They are equipped with a small burst or "pulse" of readily available energy from stored ATP, to allow most of us about thirty seconds' activity. This is the basis of sprinting, for instance, and helps explain why the 100-yard dash can be run at high speed compared with the slower pace required in distance running. After the initial burst, we require the finely tuned interaction of heart, lungs, blood vessels, and the muscle's energy stores—glycogen—to sustain our activity. This is aerobic metabolism at work.

The first thirty seconds or minute of exertion is not aerobic at all; it is *anaerobic* (without oxygen), probably a throwback to the early days of human existence when fight or flight was more necessary and the body could not wait for the necessary oxygen to reach the muscles for a response to danger. But after this burst, muscles will perform efficiently only in the presence of oxygen, burning the fuel that is stored in them from the carbohydrates we eat. During the complex breakdown of glycogen our energy supply (ATP) is renewed so long as there is enough fuel present to produce it. With enough glycogen and a substance known as *creatine phosphate* on hand in the muscles, and a well-functioning heart and set of lungs, an individual can expect to carry out vigorous physical activity for a fairly long period of time. However, all the good nourishment in the world will be of little avail if oxygen cannot be delivered in sufficient quantity to burn the fuel, as in the case of lungs diseased by smoking, or a weak heart.

When the fuel is exhausted, or when poor oxidation occurs because of heart or lung disease, a third phase takes over: *anaerobic metabolism* again. In this final phase, muscles have the ability to contract without available oxygen for a limited period of time. However, after a while lactic acid builds up, causing cramps and exhaustion. The familiar spectacle of the marathoner rubbing his/her painfully cramped leg muscles is an example of this phenomenon.

It is clear, then, that the principal means of engaging in long-term, sustained physical activity is through the use of our aerobic metabolism. Fortunately, this mechanism may be powerfully affected by training.

Training increases the efficiency of a given muscle by placing a workload on it. Muscles respond—up to a point—to stress by becoming more efficient in dealing with the stress. Unlike machine parts, which wear out with use, muscle tissue can adapt itself to the demand for more work. By training a muscle, including the heart, gradually and carefully over a period of time, its efficiency and strength can be increased many times over. A particular form of training will cause improvement up to a point, then the muscle will progress no further; if a higher load is then placed on the muscle and it is allowed to train again, an even greater degree of strength will result.

The body adapts extremely well to certain environmental conditions—to heat, cold, damp climates, altitude, activity, and inactivity. Much of our present dilemma, and one reason for writing this book, is to point out that inactivity has been endured for several generations, with disastrous consequences for the average American body. The flabbiness of muscles, including the heart, which is the end result of such a failure of physical movement, has grave consequences for health. One of the most serious, of course, is heart disease.

Training can be quite specific and in some forms does not involve the heart except in an indirect way. A great deal of weight training and isometric activity is of this kind. Strengthening an isolated muscle or group of muscles is possible through specific training techniques such as those used by the weightlifting fraternity, who pride themselves on rippling deltoids and bulging biceps.

If the heart is to be trained, it must be placed under a fairly constant level of stress for a given period of time, not too little and not too much. With its capacity to respond much like skeletal muscle, the heart can increase its efficiency, become stronger (and somewhat thicker in the bargain), thereby increasing its pumping capacity and even perhaps increasing its extraction of oxygen from the blood. A specific measure of the heart's gain in efficiency is a *drop in pulse rate for a given load*, of which we will say more shortly.

When a muscle is used under stress, it demands a greater supply of blood, which must be diverted from other organs such as the kidneys or the gastrointestinal tract. If intense use of a few muscles occurs, particularly if the heart is poorly trained, these exercises and activities—some forms of weight training, snow shoveling, pushups—may prove to be too much for the heart, resulting in undue strain or even illness. Certainly, these exercises have value for some types of work and are often used for body-building. Although, as we will point out later in reference to certain sports, they can be most valuable in conditioning for a sport, by themselves they can be dangerous and should not be undertaken in the absence of a good underlying aerobic conditioning program for the heart.

In summary, to perform exercise, particularly of the aerobic (sometimes called *endurance*) variety, a smoothly functioning oxygen delivery system must exist so that the muscles in question are well supplied. Since the aerobic sports generally require the coordinated functioning of many muscles, good heart and lung function must exist; in addition, the stress placed upon the heart by these activities results in time in the improvement of cardiac function. If heart disease is present, or chronic lung disease or smoking damage has occurred, the delivery of oxygen can be impaired and muscle glycogen will be poorly metabolized.

One principle that affects all muscles is the concept of *overload.* We have mentioned this in regard to training that places stress on the muscles. Overload is simply another way of saying that extra demands must be placed upon the muscle in order for it to improve; it implies a kind of alternating stress-rest sequence. For proper buildup of muscle strength, a specific load is placed upon a muscle, followed by a period of rest; the process is then repeated. Should a period of prolonged rest take place, deterioration in strength will occur, but this is correctable by proper training once more. At worst, the muscles will slide into a state of flabbiness—from prolonged bed rest, weightlessness (a problem thus far only for astronauts), or from embracing a sedentary life for some months.

Our heart muscles may not function at an optimal level for a variety of reasons, not all of them related to disease. The heart may work poorly as a result of improper training, advanced age, external problems like smoking or high altitude, or infections and diseases of other organs. But the main reason why so many people in this country have hearts that function poorly is because they aren't trained at all.

Cardiac training means something very specific: aerobic exercise carried out for about thirty minutes, at least three times a week, at an intensity sufficient to raise the pulse (heart) rate to a specific threshold level. This threshold level varies according to age, decreasing as age increases, and, to some extent, physical conditioning. While there is an inexorable

MAXIMAL ATTAINABLE HEART RATE AND TARGET ZONE*

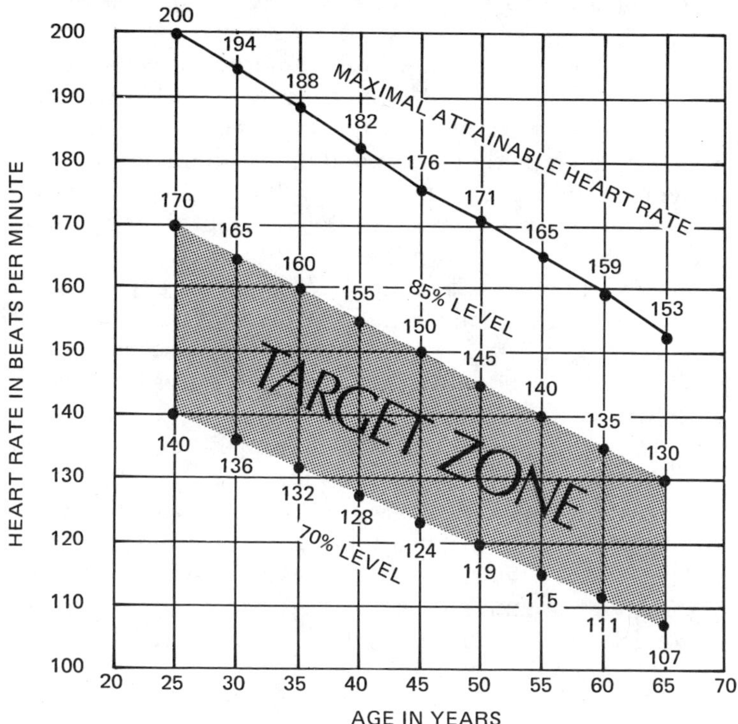

This figure shows that as we grow older, the highest heart rate which can be reached during all-out effort falls. These numerical values are "average" values for age. Note that one-third of the population may differ from these values. It is quite possible that a normal 50-year-old man may have a maximum heart rate of 195 or that a 30-year-old man might have a maximum of only 168. The same limitations apply to the 70 per cent and 85 per cent of maximum lines.

*From Lenore R. Zohman, *Beyond Diet . . . Exercise Your Way to Fitness and Heart Health* (Englewood Cliffs, N.J.: CPC International Inc., 1974), p. 15.

lessening of maximum pulse with advancing age, it is nevertheless true that a very fit elderly person can be in much better shape than a person in his/her twenties who does not exercise. In fact, it would be far better if we had some measure of *physiologic* age to which we could refer rather than strict chronological age. All of us know people in their thirties who seem quite old and "young" seventy-year-olds.

The heart rate graph will doubtless become a familiar sight in years to come; it is the exercise physiologist's standard way of looking at aerobic conditioning requirements. Since the heart rate—pulse—corresponds fairly accurately with oxygen uptake (which can't be measured without sophisticated laboratory devices), pulse is a generally accepted and convenient way of assessing your own level of conditioning.

Pulse taking isn't difficult. The preferred method is to place a moderate amount of pressure over the carotid artery in the neck, although the radial artery pulse at the wrist is certainly acceptable, as is the heart rate measured by placing your hand over the heart.

The heart rate graph, with its target zone, gives us a set of guidelines for all aerobic exercise. If a 45-year-old person, for instance, sets out after years of inactivity to exercise, a target pulse of 160 might be achieved merely with brisk walking. This is where his/her program should start, not with jogging, fast swimming, or any of the more strenuous aerobic methods, and certainly not with isometrics, which tend to drive the pulse to extremely high levels.

Your pulse should be taken as soon as you stop a phase of your exercise. Record it for ten seconds. Multiplying by six, of course, gives you the rate for one minute. The slight inaccuracies of this method (compared, say, to using a monitor or other more sophisticated method) are far outweighed by the cost and the gain in self-confidence resulting from measuring your own physiologic processes.

As training progresses, the heart in an otherwise healthy person adapts, principally because the stroke volume (the amount of blood pumped out of the heart on each stroke) becomes greater, rising to a level that can be achieved with maximum training. In other words, heart output—which in an *un*trained person can be raised only if the heart beats faster—increases in *trained* individuals because of a greater heart muscle mass and the consequent increase in the power of the pump—the heart—itself. Thus, the first step in training an individual is to train the heart itself. Athletes who do not train their hearts (weightlifters, body-builders, and football linesmen often neglect this) rank no higher than sedentary but otherwise healthy people when their aerobic power is measured.

A minimally well trained heart can usually be achieved in a matter of six to fifteen weeks, depending upon adherence to the program as well as a person's previous state of health. If the program lapses, training must revert to a lower level. On the other hand, a considerable improvement in heart function can be gained at modest cost by developing more intensity of training. However, pushing the program beyond forty-five minutes in length, or performing more than five days a week will yield little extra physiologic benefit.

One method of accomplishing a higher level of performance is called *interval* training. A typical interval training program based upon walking might go like this: walk briskly enough to ensure that the pulse has reached the target zone, pick out a landmark (a telephone pole, a house) about 100 yards ahead. Increase your pace to a very brisk walk, swinging your arms at the same time, until you reach your goal, then decelerate to your previous pace. You should have become a little winded, perhaps have worked up a light sweat, but you should not have become exhausted and should be able to continue on without difficulty.

This technique can be applied to any aerobic sports—swimming, cycling, running. Its effect is to train the heart and involve skeletal muscles to a higher level of performance, and, ultimately, if one wishes, to a competitive grade of activity.

Breathlessness is a rough measure of knowing when you have approached your limit or gone too far. The "talk test" advocated by many exercise physiologists consists simply of trying to speak while exercising. That's why it is usually a good idea to exercise with a friend who is willing to walk or run at your pace. If you can carry on a conversation with your companion, you know you haven't exceeded your aerobic capacity, that you haven't gone into serious *oxygen debt*, which you must pay back by breathing hard at the end of your exertion. If you're breathless while conversing and walking up a steep hill, slow down, adapt to a lower level of training, and look forward to the day when, fully trained, you can talk and run at the same time.

The oxygen debt is incurred during the beginning of exercise, when the brief anaerobic period mentioned earlier occurs and stored muscle energy is liberated as a burst of power. Any other anaerobic processes utilized during prolonged exercise will also contribute to this debt, which must be paid back at the end. Oxygen is needed during the recovery phase to recharge the system. After an intense period of exercise, then, there is a period of heavy breathing, which is entirely normal. The "cool-down" period recommended for all exercise allows time and attention to be devoted to this phenomenon.

Finally, it is important to understand that insofar as aerobic conditioning and caloric expenditure are concerned, the important factor is the distance covered, not the intensity of exercise. The walker who travels five miles uses as much energy as the runner who runs the same distance, although of course the runner will cover the space in a shorter time.

Recent evidence recommends a brisk walking program, carried out for about half an hour, three days a week, with the heart rate at about 50 percent of maximum oxygen capacity (which is about 60 percent of the maximum pulse for one's age). This supplies the walker with sufficient exercise to protect himself/herself effectively against heart disease, based upon data gathered from several important investigations. One study of 17,000 Harvard alumni shows that a calorie expenditure, through exercise, of 2000 cal/week, or about 300 cal/day, is sufficient to be linked with a lower incidence of heart disease. A group of London civil service workers who walked twenty minutes to and from work had a heart disease rate considerably lower than a group who didn't walk to work. These modest commitments in exercise certainly had considerable payoff.

Adding another fifteen minutes or more to the basic half-hour walking program will improve aerobic capacity to a limited degree; and the same is true if the program is extended to five days per week from three. It appears that more benefit is gained from increasing the number of days rather than increasing the daily time spent. But beyond five days, no discernible improvement can be shown.

This allows us to approach our fitness goals with considerable flexibility. Fortunately improvement in aerobic capacity can occur in *any* form of aerobic activity, and it makes no difference whether it is intermittent or continuous. Thus we can tailor a personal fitness program to our convenience.

Professor Åstrand's prescription comes closest to the mark: a daily investment of one hour of aerobic activity. This might mean walking partway to work (getting off the bus several stops from work, or parking the car farther away), walking at lunch, climbing a lot of stairs instead of taking the elevator, and so on. All of these exercises can be taken in small doses if one wishes. Sixty one-minute periods, twelve five-minute periods, four fifteen-minute periods, or one hour-long workout—it makes no difference whatsoever. The benefits are the same. In addition, Professor Åstrand recommends three intense workouts per week of about thirty minutes each. This not only reinforces the existing aerobic capacity but allows one to move toward higher ground if desired.

Because there are other reasons to do more than this relatively brief amount of exercise, there is no reason to place a lid on the activity; more might suit certain circumstances. It may be an absolute necessity if one is training for a distance run or a cycling tour in which many miles are involved. Longer exercises could have significant psychological benefits for some people. But from the standpoint of cardiovascular training and improvement, as well as the maintenance requirements of a healthy heart, the time and energy necessary are relatively modest and well within the reach of almost everyone.

The consequences of not doing this kind of activity are clearly visible all around us, at least in terms of caloric effects. A walk of 1¼ miles per day will consume 100 calories; approximately ten pounds of weight per year are thus burned off. Obesity can be thought of as the result of not walking that distance. The usual pattern, of course, in weight problems is gradual and subtle increments in weight, perhaps three or four pounds a year, until some level is reached, at which point the person affected begins an endless round of fad and starvation-like diets. Even if, as happens through good group-oriented weight-reduction programs, there is success in losing weight, there is considerable difficulty in maintaining the ideal weight if calories are not being burned off. Often the weight comes back. It is far more efficient to assist the weight-reduction process with an active, calorie-burning lifetime fitness program. The payoff, in terms of better appearance, improved health, increased work capacity, and reduction of fatigue is obvious.

The maintenance of a fitness program for improved cardiovascular performance should be a basic personal goal for everyone. Most of us exercise not because we are trying to prevent heart disease, but because we want to feel better, more in charge of our bodies, more vigorous, more alive. A well-functioning heart will help give us these feelings.

EXERCISE TESTING

One way to determine whether a person is capable of beginning an exercise program and whether a specific program is safe for that person is *exercise testing*, also called *stress testing* or *endurance testing*. Perhaps a better term for this procedure would be *exercise tolerance testing*, since the word *stress* has such a loaded meaning for so many people.

There are various reasons to have an exercise tolerance test. In our experience, extremely fit people do not need the test to attempt to screen for heart disease (one of the recognized uses of the test) but rather as a way of providing feedback to them concerning their capabilities. Since the procedure isn't cheap, its availability is limited at this time. Expansion will depend upon whether we can produce larger numbers of certified exercise testers and whether ways can be found to avoid having the highly paid physician's presence required at the test because of liability considerations.

Assuming a person is normal, wants to exercise, and is free of major risks, the test can assess aerobic capacity and assist in the formulation of an exercise prescription. If done yearly, there is also, as mentioned earlier, feedback of information to the exerciser himself/herself, providing motivation for maintenance or improvement. At times, of course, the questions asked by patients and physicians are how much exercise should a patient with known heart disease do, and how much might be beneficial in the treatment of heart disease?

Exercise testing has become scientifically sophisticated compared to the days when subjects were required to march up and down a set of two steps and pulse measurements were taken to determine a hypothetical fitness level. This was the old "Harvard Step Test" and was thoroughly despised by a generation of college freshmen who were put through their paces en masse while (it seemed) ex-Marine drill instructors held stopwatches and barked instructions.

The Step Test has given way to a more refined but more expensive laboratory approach using an ergometer, which is a device capable of being set at various workloads, employing resistance (the bicycle ergometer) or a combination of speeds and incline, with walking or running as the test exercise (the treadmill ergometer). Since ergometers can be set exactly and are calibrated exactly, repeated testing on a machine can yield important information over time. The Step Test lacked such reliability. If a person has, between tests, been swimming, running, playing tennis, or otherwise attempting to improve performance, this activity should show up on the test, measured by a pulse rate. This basic equipment can be expanded to determine whether latent heart disease might be present, with an electrocardiograph attached and a record being made while the subject is exercising.

Conditions on the treadmill or bicycle are somewhat like those encountered during exercise or physical stress in more natural settings, and if a change occurs—principally an alteration of a segment of the EKG tracing—there is a chance that the blood supply to the heart may be insufficient for such exertion. Should chest pain accompany this finding, the possibility of heart disease as the cause of exercise-induced chest pain is fairly high. In addition, irregularities of the rhythm of the heart, which occur in some persons with more frequency during exercise, can be observed and recorded. A similar technique, with additional applications beyond the exercise field, is the use of the *Holter Monitor*, which records an electrocardiogram over a number of hours with a tape recorder. This monitor and, occasionally, telemetry (remote control transmission of heartbeat) are used to assess exercise and its relationship to heartbeat irregularities.

It is well to remember that exercise testing is not a thoroughly accurate science. There are sufficiently false positive tests (indications of abnormality when none exists) and false negatives (negative results in the presence of proven disease) to make the test results subject to misinterpretation or overinterpretation. Like many other medical tests, including the electrocardiogram itself, this is simply a useful tool in the hands of the medical practitioner. Weighing all the existing evidence is necessary. Reliance upon the exercise tolerance test alone, or interpretation by inexperienced personnel, is inadvisable.

Many people who have suffered heart attacks have entered cardiac rehabilitation programs in which the basic method of treatment is exercise; often these programs are located outside hospitals, in YMCAs and similar community settings. By testing on a periodic basis, the physician can make careful observations concerning the condition of the heart as the individual becomes more and more fit. Although the evidence from these programs is still sketchy, particularly in terms of whether more lives are actually prolonged through this method, the feeling of confidence and well-being that patients report is extraordinary and could in itself justify the effort. In a number of cases, people who have had heart attacks have been trained, under special circumstances, to run very great distances, and a group of these former heart patients runs in the Boston Marathon every year.

For whom is testing best suited? Standards vary, and, as noted, cost is a major factor. Perhaps it is easier to say who does *not* require testing, at least who does not need screening for heart disease. Those of any age who have been engaged in long-term aerobic fitness programs without difficulty probably don't need testing. For example, the seventy-year-old who has jogged three times a week for years at a level sufficient to raise his/her pulse to the target rate doesn't need screening. Similarly, a young person (under the arbitrary age of thirty-five) who has been healthy and who has no risk factors—a family history of heart disease at an early age, cigarette addiction, high blood pressure, or an excessively high blood cholesterol level—doesn't need screening. Apart from these two groups, it is generally recommended that other adults—people over thirty-five who are just starting to exercise, those with significant risk factors (whatever their age), and people with known heart disease wishing to exercise—should be tested.

Should this recommendation be fully accepted, it is clear that we would not have the resources to test all those who might be eligible. At this time facilities are limited, as are the required highly trained personnel. Unfortunately, insurance companies, with few exceptions, are generally not willing to pay for the test when it is performed for purely preventive reasons.

Other countries, particularly the Scandinavian nations, have solved the problem by placing testing facilities in the community, through the cooperation of recreation departments and industry. The test—for fitness testing purposes only, not cardiac screening—is administered by a nonmedical but well-trained, certified exercise professional. This takes considerable pressure off the medical profession, which can then devote its time and energies to testing those with possible, or established heart disease.

Whatever the purpose of testing, whether to find out if the heart is functioning at a low level in a healthy person or whether it is in fact affected by disease, the testing will produce information on which basis the exercise program is to be drawn up, unless there is some contraindication to exercise. By combining data from the test with the person's own likes and dislikes, a set of activities can be suggested that will be safe and that will assist in the development of a stronger heart and skeletal muscles. The exercise itself—walking, swimming, or whatever is desirable—is specified. Appropriate warm-up and cool-down phases of five to ten minutes are listed. Next, a target heart rate is specified. Then, the frequency of participation is given: usually a minimum of three days a week and thirty minutes for each session. Longer sessions can be suggested if obesity is a problem. Finally, a list of cautions and suggestions about prevention of injuries is provided.

Obviously there is a need to make this test more readily available, at low cost, so that the important question how fit am I now? can be answered for Americans. Nothing now available approaches the low cost—the equivalent of $10 to $15—which the Swedes pay in their community-based Trim Centers. A fascinating and as yet unexplored area for investigation about the exercise test is its role in motivation. Almost everyone who administers the test is impressed with how effective a first test is in giving people the psychological boost they seem to need to begin exercising. Many of these same people want to come back for yearly tests to assess their progress.

HOW SAFE IS EXERCISE?

Almost everyone has heard some story about a person who dies while jogging, presumably from a cardiac arrest. It does little good to cite statistics about the larger chance everyone has of being hit by an automobile. If you do that, your friends will tell you about some jogger who was struck by an automobile.

Testing does have a limited but important role to play

here. Screening can bring out abnormalities that might become dangerous during exercise. Generally speaking, people with fainting spells, particularly during exercise, and those with cardiac murmurs of certain types (particularly the mitral systolic click-murmur syndrome, which has been known to occur in conjunction with rhythm disturbances, chest pain, and fainting spells and which should be looked for in young athletes) should be examined more extensively than the average person.

But for the rest of us exercise testing will not screen for the extremely rare occurrence of heart trouble *brought on* by exercise. As Professor Åstrand has remarked, not altogether facetiously, it makes more sense to test those who plan to have a sedentary life than those who are starting an exercise program, since the former are at much more risk of heart disease.

Cautions

There are some well-recognized cautions, the first of which is do not overdo anything. If you're like many Americans, you wish to excel. But try to keep things in perspective. Remember there is always someone who can train longer and harder than you—or who is younger and has the ability and/or stamina to outdo you much of the time. It's yourself against whom you should compete: that is, how much farther, or faster, did you go compared with the last time? Or did you add another half mile to your swimming laps so that you'll make fifty miles by the end of the summer? In order to stay within safe limits, you should not exceed your own aerobic capacity. This may require adding introspection and moderation to your sporting activities.

Remember that walking, the basis of all other aerobic work, is safe and highly beneficial; almost no one gets cardiac problems while walking, unless he/she is already crippled by heart disease. Swimming, too, can be a prudent beginning (as well as advanced) life sport. As long as your stroke is efficient, starting with a slow pace will be safe and beneficial.

Second, do not, under any circumstances, engage in moderate to heavy aerobic work when you have a fever or other sign of infection. There is an increased sensitivity of the heart muscle to injury during some infections, particularly those caused by viruses, some of which seem to have a capacity to injure the tissue.

Third, do not exercise heavily just after eating. Your stomach and intestines need the blood and have a hard time sharing it with your heart and muscles.

Fourth, avoid exercising in extremes of temperature unless you are in top condition and are prepared to make the necessary adjustments—fluid replacement in hot weather or cold protection in winter conditions—to maintain your health under these conditions. These topics will be discussed in chapter five.

Finally, and equally important, make exercising fun. Even though we have spent a lot of time talking about how to make your heart healthy, most of us don't run or swim or play sports because we are trying to stave off heart disease. We are active in order to get outdoors, expand our territory, think and feel better, and, above all, achieve a sense of control over our bodies. Running, swimming, dancing, hiking, walking, cycling—all allow us to expand our culturally imposed physiologic limits. (Of course we wouldn't need to do this if our lives were spent foraging for vegetables and hunting animals.) Most of us have a need to counter the effects of inactivity. If at the same time we add an understanding of what our body is doing to our enjoyment of movement, we make the experience more intense and rewarding. The burden of being sedentary will have been replaced with a new sense of pleasure in strength, endurance, and control.

3. Training Your Muscles and Joints

IT IS becoming increasingly evident that safe athletic conditioning must include techniques for improving the strength, endurance, and flexibility of the muscles and the strength of the bone, ligaments and cartilage. Too often, a carefully planned program is aborted because of a pulled hamstring, Achilles' tendinitis, or fracture of the leg. While training objectives of the distance runner and body-builder are different, both must use sound principles of muscle training.

Why lift weights? If you are thinking of, or already participating in some highly aerobic sport like swimming, cycling, or running, you might look askance at weightlifting. Isn't that for the musclebound crowd, sweating and groaning away in some basement full of chrome junk?

Weight training does have a place, nevertheless. Its function, we feel, is not to improve the appearance of the body, but rather to increase the structural strength of the bones, ligaments, and tendons of the arms, legs, and back, thereby rendering them more resistant to injury while participating in sports. The common "tennis elbow" of racquet sports, the "pulled hamstring" of the weekend soccer or football player, or the abused knee ligaments of the recreational basketball player can be prevented by proper weight training. The fear that the muscles being stressed in weight training will cause the participant to become a grotesque caricature of the human form can be dismissed. Proper weight training, as outlined here, serves only to allow the muscles to move more smoothly, since their supporting structures have been stretched and relaxed to allow them to do so.

PRINCIPLES: SPECIFICITY, OVERLOAD, AND REST

Any fitness or strengthening program should be specifically designed for particular demands to be placed on the body. A highly trained gymnast may be a totally unfit soccer player, or distance cyclist. Back muscles that can tolerate eight hours of canoeing may complain after a vigorous set of tennis.

The human body responds to external stress by changing its structure in such a way as to decrease the chance of injury to itself. For example, if you lift a weight a number of times, your body will increase the size and strength of the muscles, tendons, ligaments, and bones of your arm to prevent injury from the weight. If, on the other hand, the body senses no threat to itself or its structures from the weight, i.e., the weight is too "light," no increase in strength will occur.

This protective mechanism of the body to adapt its structure, and to some extent its function, to imposed demands occurs not only in the muscles and bones but also in the heart, lungs, and other organs and body systems. The body's response to systematic running is to increase both the amount of blood pumped by the heart and the air inspired by the lungs, as well as to strengthen the bones, muscles, and ligaments of the legs. Again, the intensity of exercise must be sufficient to "overload" the structural elements and yet not so much as to cause injury to these structures.

If overload stress is followed by a period of rest, so that the body has sufficient time to reinforce itself, a progressive increase in fitness or, in the case of the muscles, strength, will occur.

Though training and conditioning are often done primarily to improve athletic skill, the strengthening of muscles and bones that results from training also protects the body from injury. Any improvement in athletic performance is, from the body's point of view, totally coincidental.

Improved fitness is obtained from alternating overload and

rest; too much overload or too little rest can result in injury. Conversely, too little overload or too much rest will not condition or strengthen the body, nor reduce the chance of injury from a sport.

It is useful to divide musculoskeletal conditioning into these three areas: (1) muscle conditioning, (2) conditioning of the structural elements of bone ligaments and cartilage, and (3) flexibility training.

MUSCLE CONDITIONING

There are two primary elements to consider in a muscle-conditioning program: the demands that the particular sport will place upon one's muscle and the facilities or techniques available for training.

Sport analysis is in its infancy in this country. However, there have been some studies using high-speed cinematography, force plates, and cable tensiometers in such sports as weight-lifting, gymnastics, and running that have helped to determine the particular muscles used and the duration of their use. These studies indicate also the type of muscle contraction and the intensity required. More frequently, the coach or athlete must assess the musculoskeletal demands of a particular sport and design training programs that will enable the athlete to meet these demands, avoid injury, and improve performance.

To better understand muscle training, it is necessary to know a little about the structure of the muscles and how they work. Each skeleton muscle is made up of two types of tissue: the contractile fibers in the body of the muscle and the connective tissue sheaths and fibers extending through the muscle and converging to form the tendons on each end of the muscle. Skeletal muscles are connected to bone directly by their tendons and span the joints of the body. When an electrical impulse travels down a motor nerve, it is transmitted to the muscle. This causes a contraction of the muscle, and force is exerted at the bony insertions.

While each muscle fiber responds to an electrical stimulus in only one way, i.e., by shortening itself a fixed distance, the total force delivered by the muscle depends on a number of factors, including the percentage of the total muscle fibers of the muscle contracting, the coordination of these contractions, and the position of the joint at the time the muscle contracts.

Strength and Endurance

A number of researchers have found that muscle fibers, when viewed under a high-power electron microscope, show different chemical and metabolic characteristics. There are two types of fibers, *fast-twitch* and *slow-twitch.*

Fast-twitch fibers have a large supply of high-energy phosphates, mostly in the form of ATP. Apparently, people with a high percentage of fast-twitch fibers tend to do well in sprintlike activities but do not have the capacity for endurance work. Conversely, those with an abundance of slow-twitch fibers appear to have the mechanism to carry out long-term activities requiring very efficient oxidative metabolism. This would apply, for instance, to middle-distance running, swimming, or games like basketball or soccer. Unfortunately, this knowledge can be obtained only from muscle biopsy—a painful procedure. Thus the knowledge is limited to research technique at this time, though it has potentially great significance for the understanding of human performance.

While *muscle strength* is usually described as the maximal force that a muscle group can exert against the resistance in a single effort, it most frequently is determined as the maximal amount of weight that can be moved through a full range of motion by a muscle group. *Muscle endurance,* on the other hand, is the ability of the muscle group to perform repeated contractions or to maintain a single contraction for an extended period of time. While an increase in both muscle strength and endurance will result from most training programs, the way in which the muscle work is performed, or the program design, can favor one or the other aspect of muscle conditioning.

There are actually four different ways in which muscular activity can be performed by the body, and programs of muscle training that primarily utilize one or another type of these muscle activities have been developed. They are isometric, isokinetic, dynamic concentric, and dynamic eccentric.

In an *isometric* contraction, there is no actual movement of the skeletal elements or shortening of the muscle despite the development of maximal force by the muscle. ("Charles Atlas" types of muscle-building use isometric contractions, as does the so-called Bullworker.) Several important points must be made about isometric strength-training programs. While significant increases in strength and muscle bulk can result from an isometric program, there is not a great improvement in endurance. In addition, strength development depends on the joint angle at which the isometric work is performed. A muscle group may gain significant strength at one particular joint position yet remain relatively weak at other positions that have not been trained.

There are, however, certain real advantages to isometric exercises. They can be done without much equipment. By using the opposite arm or leg for resistance, or one's own desk or chair at work, most of the major muscle groups can be given an isometric workout. In addition, rehabilitation of an injured arm or leg is often most effectively carried out by beginning with isometric exercises that can be done progressively and painlessly. (Beginning with dynamic exercises, in which there is movement of the joint, can result in pain and further disability.) Such conditions as "runners' knee" respond best to an isometric leg-strengthening program, at least at first.

It is well to remember that injury can result from isometric exercises improperly done. Buildup of force should be gradual—with maximum force held for no more than seven to ten seconds. Proper position of the body before beginning is important to avoid back, neck, or shoulder injuries. Joint positions should be changed each time to get the most strengthening through the range of motions of the muscle.

Ideally, an isometric exercise program should include three to five different repetitions done at various positions in the joints and held for a duration of seven to ten seconds each.

The three other types of muscle action are all known as *dynamic* (as opposed to *isometric*). They are *eccentric*, *concentric*, and *isokinetic*. No matter what kind you choose, or which is best for you, you will hear frequent mention of the terms *repetition*, *set*, and *frequency* (of training) in connection with these activities.

A *repetition* is the performance of a given weight-training exercise. A *set* is the performance of a particular number of repetitions of the same exercise. *Frequency* refers, of course, to the number of times per week that an exercise set should be repeated.

Usually a frequency of not more than every other day for weight-training exercises is recommended to give the body time to rebuild itself after the stress of a session and thus increase the strength of each muscle group being trained. For this reason, daily performance of weight training is not recommended. On the "rest" day, however, some aerobic activity, like a distance swim or run might be carried out. Such activities place a very different kind of demand on the body, thus keeping the cardiovascular system at top efficiency.

Sets will vary depending upon the specific goals of a program. One recommendation might be a single set of three to five repetitions; another might be three sets of seven to ten repetitions of each exercise. In most cases, weight training requires expert guidance and any organization sponsoring such a program should have qualified instructors available.

The most common type of dynamic exercise is *concentric* activity, in which the muscles are shortened as movement takes place. This technique of muscle training is used by both major systems of weight training: the free-weight system, which uses barbells or dumbbells, and certain exercise machines that use weights and pulleys, such as the Universal Gym or Nautilus systems. Then again, exercises that use only the body weight as resistance, such as situps or pushups, are also dynamic concentric exercises.

Each system has its die-hard advocates. Free-weight systems are much less expensive than machines and thus more generally available. With some of the lifts, such as the bench press, however, there should be a second person present to hold or guide you in situations of potential injury (referred to as "spotting"). A sudden twist can throw you off balance and seriously injure a muscle or ligament. The machines are designed to limit the chance of injury. In particular, Nautilus machines are conceived to protect the back while you are performing the exercises. Also, strengthening is specifically limited to an isolated group of muscles and the joints are put through a full range of motion with each repetition.

Using free weights or the machines, you may use either a high-repetition or a low-repetition program of weight training. Low-repetition programs, with one to three repetitions, are used to increase strength or muscle size, while high-repetition programs, using up to thirty repetitions, have been recommended for increased endurance.

Since a combination of muscle strength and endurance is ideal for most sports, a program that incorporates both is recommended. Studies have shown that the best results are obtained by weightlifting programs using the maximum weight that can be lifted seven to ten times. For free weights or the Universal Gym, two or three separate sets of seven to ten repetitions each is recommended, with exercises alternating between the arms and legs. With the Nautilus system, a single set of seven to ten repetitions on each machine is recommended.

There has been an increased interest recently in *eccentric* or "negative work" techniques of weight training, in which the muscle being used is actually being lengthened as it contracts. Here, external resistance exceeds the force the muscle can develop and the muscle is progressively lengthened while it attempts to develop maximal tension. Much of the muscle activity in running is eccentric, for instance, as when the hamstrings are actively contracting to decelerate the leg at the end of the stride. Here the hamstrings, while actively contracting to resist the forward movement of the leg, are being progressively lengthened.

When using free weights, or the Universal Gym for negative work, an assistant, or "spotter," is usually required to help position the weights or bars for maximum benefit.

In *isokinetic* techniques of weight training, the muscle contracts at a fixed rate of speed, resulting in a constant torque throughout the range of motion. Although much investigation is now being done on isokinetic types of exercises, their role in basic strength training remains to be determined.

No matter what system of muscle strengthening is used, the basic principles of safe training are the same. You must understand the technique of performing each lift or maneuver and position your body to eliminate the possibility of injury—particularly to the back or shoulders. Sufficient resistance or weight must be used to stress the muscles or no increases in strength will be obtained. Furthermore, studies of low-weight high-repetition programs have shown that for muscle endurance and strength there is no particular advantage over programs of seven to ten repetitions. On the other hand, the use of excessive weights should be avoided. With heavy weights, even using only two to three repetitions, the risk of injury is increased and little improvement in muscle endurance occurs. Finally, it is important to remember that the exercise should be performed slowly and evenly to decrease the chance of injury and take full advantage of both the concentric and eccentric benefits.

An exercise session of one to three sets of seven to ten repetitions per set, with particular emphasis on the muscles most used in the target sport, performed once a day on alternate days, will maximize increases in muscle strength while minimizing the potential for injury. The amount of weight lifted is progressively increased as strength increases, while the number of repetitions remains between seven and ten.

CONDITIONING THE BONES

The components of the musculoskeletal system (bones, ligaments and cartilege) will undergo structural changes in response to repeated stress. Simply running on a level surface delivers shock waves with a force of two to three times the body weight to the legs and feet.

If such stress is done at a rate that allows the body tissue time to adjust properly, the size of the bones and the ligaments of the lower extremities will increase and their internal structure will be reinforced. The end result is strength development. This will also be seen in the upper extremities. X-rays show that the pitching arm of the baseball player and the serving arm of the tennis player have larger and heavier bones than the players' less active arms.

It is important to realize that the first stage in this process involves absorbing certain parts of the preexisting bone before the newer reinforcing elements of bone are added. At this stage of reabsorption, the bone may actually be weaker than it was before training began. Slow, progressive training techniques, which increase the stress applied to the arms or legs, are very important to permit the body to both remodel old bone and form newer, stronger bony elements. If this is not done, the weakened bone may actually fracture.

The time required for proper training of the bones and ligaments will depend on a number of factors in a given athlete, including age, size, previous training, relative flexibility and strength of the muscles and tendons, and, in running, the type of shoe worn and the training surface. While it takes much longer to gain skeletal fitness than it does to develop muscular and cardiac fitness, it is also probable that skeletal fitness is lost less rapidly than the other two types.

The key factor in training and toughening the bones and ligaments is the rate at which training is done, as measured by total distance per running session and total distance per week or month. As an example, for the adult novice runner, we generally recommend increasing distance by no more than one to two miles per week, with increases of no more than a quarter of a mile per running session.

Increased distance per week should not exceed 10 percent of the previous week. Thus, a runner doing thirty miles per week would not increase her/his mileage by more than three miles per week, with the total increase spread over four to six running sessions. To advance more rapidly might well result in one or another overuse syndrome (see chapter five).

FLEXIBILITY TRAINING

Perhaps the area of conditioning that has received the least attention until quite recently has been flexibility and flexibility training. Even in sports such as gymnastics, dance, figure skating, and swimming, where limberness or flexibility is an important part of basic technique, individuals with exceptional flexibility have frequently excelled, but the systematic use of flexibility or stretching exercises for all participants has been generally neglected. It has recently been documented that proper stretching and flexibility exercises can help improve athletic performance and prevent injuries in sports as diverse as football, distance running, and racquetball.

Flexibility is the range of motion attainable in a given joint. The three factors affecting flexibility are the bony "fit" of the two or more bones making up the joint, the tightness of the ligaments of the joint, and thirdly, the flexibility of the muscle/tendon units spanning the joint. Recent studies have put to rest the myth that strong muscles are "tight" and that the "loose" athlete is weaker. But prohibitions against football players swimming during the season and swimmers lifting weights can still be heard. A well-balanced training program results in both flexible and strong muscle/tendon units and ligaments.

Proper flexibility in an athlete helps prevent injury in at least three ways: (1) the supple muscle/tendon unit is less prone to tears or sprains caused by stretch, (2) the chance of ligament sprain, joint dislocation, or even fracture from a given movement is decreased because the flexible joint has an increased range, and (3) supple muscle/tendon units put less strain on adjacent joints in the course of a given athletic movement. An athlete with tight hamstrings is not only at increased risk of injury to the tight muscles themselves ("pulled hamstrings"), but he/she also puts increased stress upon the lower back, hips, and knees because of the tight muscles.

There are three stretching techniques in common use: fast, slow, and the so-called facilitative. *Ballistic*, or *fast stretching*, in which a series of bounces or rapid stretches are applied to the muscles, has been used for many years and is most familiar in such time-honored military exercises as toe touches, squat thrusts, and jumping jacks. Though these exercises may be useful as part of precompetition warm-up to raise a light sweat and increase blood flow to the muscle, there is evidence now that they do little to permanently increase flexibility, and may actually make the muscle/tendon units tighten. In addition, injury to the muscle, tendons, and even ligaments can result, particularly if a major portion of the upper body weight is used in the bounce.

Slow stretch technique gradually lengthens the ligaments and muscle/tendon units and holds them at their elongated position for a variable period of time. It has been shown to be effective in increasing both short-term flexibility (as in a warm-up before competition) and in increasing or maintaining flexibility over the long term as part of a regular exercise program. It is important to remember that muscle soreness can result from holding the stretch too long. Usually the best pattern to follow is a series of two to four separate stretches held ten to twenty seconds for each muscle group being stretched.

Relaxation is essential to slow stretch technique. The value of this in conditions as diverse as cerebral palsy and childbirth has been proven. The brain and spinal cord are constantly sending out stimulatory and inhibitory signals to the muscles, and thus they too contribute to muscle tone. It is vital to the success of the slow stretch technique that a conscious effort be made to relax the entire body in addition to the particular muscle or muscle group being worked on; only in this way will a fully relaxed muscle develop. Our psychic control mechanisms play a major role in the stressing and relaxing of muscles; most of us spend our days under the kind of pressure that, while it heightens muscle tone, does not sufficiently relax muscles.

Facilitative stretching is an extension of the slow stretch technique in which additional reflexes are used to further relax the already lengthened structures and to allow further elongation. In this technique, a slow stretch is applied to the primary structures. After maintaining the fully stretched position for five to ten seconds, the primary muscles being stretched are isometrically contracted for five to ten seconds, and then further elongated. The combination of stretch and isometric contraction is repeated until pain develops. This sequence adapts the muscle to function at an increased length. The major drawback is that it usually requires an experienced assistant to maintain joint position during the isometric contraction and to gently assist in obtaining the further stretched position. Serious injury may result if the assistant attempts to push during the successive stretching.

Sport Specific Stretching

While it is now evident that a good general flexibility program must be a part of all fitness training, certain specific stretches are particularly important in certain sports, either because of the unique requirements of the sport or because certain of the repetitive activities of the sport tend to induce tightness or lack of flexibility, in particular ligaments and muscles. We are familiar with the susceptibility of hockey players to groin pulls, and preventive stretching of the groin muscles is essential in this sport. Similarly, the thrower or server tends to develop tight muscles and ligaments in the back of the shoulder and to become loose in the front of the shoulder. Specific shoulder internal-rotation stretching exercises to combat this tendency should be done to prevent shoulder injury. We include these specifics in the chapters in this book on each lifetime sport. Further detailed information appears in the Appendix.

4. Eating for Fitness

IT ISN'T necessary to conduct an expensive new survey to determine whether we as a nation suffer from obesity—and it really is a form of suffering, in spite of what the occasional "I like me fat" groups may say. Take a careful look around you—at your fellow workers, at people you see in the street, at yourself in a mirror—you can make the diagnosis easily. Furthermore, even when obesity isn't the problem, poor nutrition often is, in spite of our advanced food technology and distribution methods and (for most of us) the ability to afford a well-balanced diet.

Although we may eat poorly, the yearning for information about food seems almost endless. Yet more confusion exists on this subject than almost any other. In fact, there continues to be a kind of persistent, puritanical myth that in order for a diet to be good for you, it must taste terrible. Food advertising in America has done little to improve the public's image of the balanced diet, nor has it emphasized the way food and exercise are intertwined.

Food faddism and weird beliefs are part of the mythology of sports as well. The early Greek athletes lived on a vegetarian diet until Eurymenes of Samos decided, in 520 B.C., that if animals could run fast, so might humans who ate their flesh. His disciple, Milo of Croton, is said to have consumed as much as twenty pounds of it a day. These athletes had no way of knowing that the requirement for protein is not that large, nor that meat is a relatively inefficient way of obtaining it, nor that protein is the *last* substance used for energy—after carbohydrates and fats. Yet our athletic training table, groaning under its burden of thick steaks, is the legacy of that belief. Some coaches—as a recent survey of Big Ten schools showed—possess some of the most bizarre convictions imaginable when it comes to food and try to foist their beliefs on their teams in the hopes that vitamin or protein supplements, or pregame pancakes, waffles, ice cream, candy bars, and even beer will supply the winning edge. Just as important as the coach's development of a higher level of nutritional understanding is the need for a better understanding of exercise physiology by dietitians and others who work in the field of nutrition. What sports need most of all is useful advice, not magic.

For the country as a whole, major changes in diet are in order, changes that have the potential for a significant impact on fitness. Such changes are not impossible. Most of us don't view ourselves in a historical perspective, but if we look at the alterations in living and eating patterns just within this century, we might be surprised. Most people believe, for instance, that the predominance of obesity in the United States is due to overeating. In one sense it is. But in fact, calorie consumption on a per capita basis has *decreased* slightly since 1910. Why all the overweight then? It's because the other side of the energy equation—expenditure—has decreased even more sharply. Even though a clerk might be eating as little as 2000 calories a day, he/she is burning up less than that by sitting at a desk and riding to work in an automobile or on the subway. A surplus of 3500 calories equals a gain of one pound. If 3500 surplus calories are eaten every two weeks, an individual will gain twenty-six pounds a year. It's not uncommon for someone who moves from an active life, of the teen years, into a sedentary occupation to gain almost that much in a year. After that, it's a constant battle to keep the weight even at that level.

A lot of people have become rich by writing and promoting books about one sort of diet or another, or by selling products promising weight reduction. That's simply an index of how many unhappy, overweight people there are. Furthermore, Americans, by subjecting themselves to starvation-level diets for intervals, tend to deprive themselves of essential nutrients that are hard to come by in diets of less than 2000 calories a day. Thus the overweight, poorly-nourished individual is a peculiarly American phenomenon.

That wasn't always so. It's only recently that we have shifted our carbohydrate intake toward sugars rather than complex starches, which are more nourishing and were once a staple part of the diet. Unlike sugars, the complex starches can be stored for energy. Sugar's main contribution is to fool the body into being less hungry while contributing absolutely no nutrition. Furthermore, sugar does a superb job of rotting teeth.

In addition, fat consumption has risen by about 30 percent since 1910. Fat, while to some degree available for energy, is stored when not needed. This is useful, if your intention is to take a trip across the desert and you have no room to store food—and if you're a camel. Unfortunately, we humans haven't found a way to store fat energy as efficiently as those animals. Fat makes it hard for the human body to do its job of movement, since we lack the camel's hump, which is placed much like a pack frame on its back. Human fat just gets in the way and becomes unsightly.

The drop in our consumption of fresh fruit, wheat flour, fresh potatoes and vegetables within the past several generations has been offset by an explosion of intake of sugar, beef, poultry, corn syrup, soft drinks, and fast foods. While it is possible to make a balanced diet out of the choices available (even fast foods), the sad fact is that we Americans have moved to a remote sector of the food spectrum, causing us to become among the most bizarre eaters in human history. Some future anthropologist who digs up our shards and excavates our dwellings may well wonder whether the diet we lived on was the cause of our decline.

Because our diet has become so unhealthy, a congressional committee, the Senate Select Committee on Nutrition and Human Needs, after exhaustive hearings, recommended a number of revisions in the national diet. These changes, set forth in the committee's 1977 report, would have a positive impact on the nation's health, particularly in the prevention of cardiovascular disease.

The dietary goals offered by the committee are as follows:

1. *To avoid overweight, consume only as much energy (calories) as needed; if overweight, decrease caloric intake and increase exercise.*
2. *Increase the consumption of complex carbohydrates and "naturally occurring" sugars from about 28 percent (the present level) to about 48 percent of caloric intake.*

   Fruits, vegetables, and grains, including breads and pasta, as well as starchy vegetables, are in these groups. Such carbohydrates are necessary for vigorous physical activity, since they are stored as glycogen in our muscles (see chapter two) to be oxidized for energy during muscle contraction. By eating this type of carbohydrate, your body consumes fewer calories—too often supplied by fats and processed sugars—and obtains a high level of fiber, which is known to be necessary for proper bowel function. (Studies of various high-fiber and low-fiber diets around the world by Professor Denis Burkitt have led to the conclusion that cancer of the colon is associated with lack of fiber.)

   Complex carbohydrates are the right substance to use in a quest for lower weight, since they contain only four calories per gram, as contrasted with nine per gram in fat. (Processed sugars provide no nutrient value at all: their calories, when not needed by the body, wind up as fat.) The nutrient value of complex carbohydrates is high, their efficiency as an energy source is great, they are universally available, many can be grown in home gardens or made cheaply at home—like bread—and generally, they are economical.
3. *Reduce the consumption of refined and processed sugars by about 45 percent to account for about 10 percent of total caloric intake.*

   In other words, change the preferences of millions of Americans from soft drinks, candy, and sugared cereals toward more nutritious substances. The label on food products will tell you, in relative terms, how much sugar (as glucose, dextrose, fructose, corn syrup, honey, dextrin, molasses, etc.) is present; if sugar is one of the first three items listed, there is a lot. The benefits of lowering your sugar intake are extensive: fewer trips to the dentist (quite a financial saving there), less obesity, a healthy appetite, and a body receiving a healthier supply of other nutrients that might otherwise have been pushed out of the way by sugar.

Since so much advertising is designed to lure children into eating candylike breakfast substances (it's hard to describe them as cereals, for many of them have more sugar than grain), it is particularly important to encourage the children you know to eat fewer sweets, to understand their own nutritional needs, and to stop associating candy with love and affection. It's always worth looking at foods to see if this additive—a relatively new presence in our long dietary history—is present. The average American, consuming his/her annual quota of thirty-one gallons of soft drinks, appears to be due for a change.

Another source of "empty" calories is alcohol, which affects the diet much the way sugar does. Because of its depressant effect upon the central nervous system, alcohol has no place in any fitness program. However, a single drink can be a pleasant accompaniment to an after-sports get-together.

4. *Reduce overall fat consumption from the present 40 percent to about 30 percent of total calories.*

Since fat yields nine calories per gram, more than twice the caloric contribution of carbohydrates or proteins, a high intake of fats tends to fatten people—it's really that simple, though the metabolic

ALCOHOL EQUIVALENTS

One 12-oz. bottle of beer=5 oz. table wine=1½ oz. "hard" liquor.

Each of these drinks raises the blood alcohol level by about 20 mg per 100 ml of blood.

Intoxication

Quantity of Whiskey	Blood Level	Level of Intoxication
1–3 oz.	80 mg alcohol/100 ml of blood	Judgment and concentration impaired
6 oz.	100 mg/100 ml	Muscular incoordination
12 oz.	200 mg/100 ml	Speech impairment
15 oz.	300 mg/100 ml	Unconsciousness
30 oz.	400–500 mg/100 ml	Death

steps between are not. The committee's recommendation of 30 percent is thought by many to be too generous; people could easily afford to get along with 20 percent and might be even healthier as a result.

Fats have an essential role, as carriers of certain vitamins and suppliers of essential fatty acids; in addition, the body's cells have fatty constituents that must be replaced. However, our bodies don't need to store excess fat in the wrong places. Obesity is a contributing factor to high blood pressure and diabetes, and thus has a role in heart disease.

Most people don't realize how ubiquitous fat is in our diet. Cheap oils like coconut and palm, which have the disadvantage of being saturated fats, are present in coffee whiteners, cake mixes, cookies, crackers, and many other foods. Labels on these products are not much help, since the term "vegetable oil" means either saturated or unsaturated fats.

5. *Reduce saturated fat consumption to account for about 10 percent of total caloric intake, and balance that with polyunsaturated and monounsaturated fats, which should account for about 10 percent of caloric intake each.*

In addition to the vegetable oils mentioned above, other saturated fats like butter, lard, meat and chicken fat, and cheeses can raise the cholesterol level in the blood. Cholesterol has long been recognized as a risk factor in heart disease. Recent studies in Finland and Belgium, where intake of saturated fats has always been high, have shown that the associated high heart disease rate has been lowered through community-wide changes in the consumption of these fats.

The mechanism by which fats exert their influence upon the heart remains a mystery, but we know that substances like fats and cholesterol are associated with an increase of cholesterol in the bloodstream. For reasons we don't yet understand, this substance plays a part in the development of deposits in certain major blood vessels. If those vessels supplying the heart with blood—the coronary arteries—become narrowed, oxygen cannot move as efficiently to the heart muscle. Pain or impaired heart action may result, as may a blockage causing death of the heart muscle supplied by the vessel in question. This is known as a *myocardial infarction*, or, in lay terms, a heart attack.

Reduce cholesterol consumption to about 300 milligrams a day.

Controversies about cholesterol have raged for many years. Since the advent of margarine, powerful forces, representing on one hand the dairy industry (which markets cholesterol in the form of milk, butter, and cream) and on the other the margarine and vegetable oil producers, have battled over whether cholesterol is a dangerous substance. Since it is easily measured in the blood, it has become a kind of symbol for dietary-related problems, though of course it isn't the only one and may in fact not be very important, according to some experts.

Cholesterol intake averages about 700 milligrams a day in men and 500 in women, with wide variations. Aside from the sources mentioned above, a big contributor is egg yolk. Most recommendations begin with a lowering of the egg intake to perhaps two to four *visible* eggs a week (eggs find their way into a number of other foods).

Cholesterol in the bloodstream may be a useful index of the trend in a society to develop heart disease, since many countries with low rates of the disease are also characterized by having blood cholesterol levels below those found in countries like the United States or Finland. As these levels rise, as they have begun to in Japan, the medical profession and the government express concern and programs to change the diet are introduced.

A new and interesting finding concerning fats is that while the cholesterol level may be important, the level of various kinds of *lipoproteins*—chemical substances that combine with fats in the blood to transport and metabolize them—may be more important. These molecules, known as very low density lipoproteins (VLDL), low density lipoproteins (LDL), and high density lipoproteins (HDL), are related in very different ways to the development of heart disease. A preponderance of LDL and VLDL has been found to be linked with an increased risk of the disorder, while elevated levels of HDL correlate with a lowered incidence. From a practical point of view, one can raise levels of HDL and lower levels of LDL and VLDL by eating fish frequently in place of meat, exercising consistently, and—surprisingly—having a daily glass of beer or wine.

What is a high cholesterol level? Some laboratories use a figure of 250 or 300 milligrams per 100 milliliters of blood as the safe upper limit, but in other parts of the world that would seem excessively high. It should be understood that the test is not always terribly accurate, that variations from laboratory to laboratory exist, and that the test result can be a reflection of what was eaten at a recent meal. There is a general swing toward the encouragement of lowered levels—some say the highest desirable level is 220 mg/100 ml, some say 200. Since the average in a vegetarian society might be in the low 100's, there is obviously room for improvement. Heart disease, a dismal fact of life and death for millions in northern, developed countries, didn't even appear as an important statistic at the turn of the century. It now accounts for over half of all deaths in the United States.

Clearly our blood cholesterol need not be as high as it is. The Bushmen of the Kalahari desert, for instance, have levels that never top 70 mg/100 ml. While they are probably at the extreme end of cholesterol levels, so far as can be determined this seems to have no adverse effect upon their health.

As far as saturated fats and cholesterol are concerned, then, what seems to be necessary is a prudent but determined effort to considerably reduce our intake and to use physical activity to further change the ratio of "bad" to "good" lipoproteins in the bloodstream.

7. *Limit the intake of sodium by reducing the intake of salt to about five grams per day.* Most of us take in more salt than this, in processed foods, snacks, and added table salt.

Apart from its harmful effects, the use of salt more than anything else is a comment upon our lack of taste differentiation. Salt is necessary in extremely small amounts—it is an essential part of the diet—but not in the quantities used by many people. Large amounts of this chemical compound cause flooding of the taste apparatus, crowding out everything else, so that subtle flavors or the real taste of food or spices is forced underground. Most of us, if we eat a lot of potato chips, pretzels, crackers, or processed foods, simply can't taste our food. It seems to take most heavy salt users a while—weeks, perhaps—after cutting down to begin to appreciate other tastes. Since there are hundreds of different spices—most of them harmless—to choose from (other cultures have known this for centuries), stopping heavy salt intake and exploring a variety of spices can be a gratifying experience.

Excessive salt use is known to aggravate fluid-retention, which relates to liver disease and heart failure. People with these conditions know all too well how sensitive the body is to the addition of a little

salt, for the body will gain several pounds in a few hours if too much salt is used. In order to keep the body's salt-to-water ratio stable, in the presence of excess salt that cannot be normally metabolized, water is retained. This brings the dilution to a more normal level but causes the uncomfortable bloating that is characteristic of these diseases.

In addition, there is some evidence that persons who are habitual heavy users of salt from an early age are more likely to develop high blood pressure. It has been suspected for years that dietary salt reduction may have beneficial effects upon high blood pressure. Since the body's actual requirement for salt is only about 5 percent of the five grams recommended in this dietary goal, it makes good sense to hold back the salt shaker and to read the labels of packaged foods, many of which have a large amount of salt dumped in during the manufacturing process.

The dietary goals of the committee are meant as guidelines, not absolutes; they will undoubtedly be debated hotly for years, since there are articulate and knowledgeable spokespersons on all sides of the recommendations. Certainly there are wide differences between many food scientists and the food industry. Nevertheless, it is clear that health, nutrition, and physical fitness cannot be considered separately.

If you're involved in a sports program, you can't help being more attentive to the food you eat. You're doing something positive for your body by exercising, so it is illogical to tear it down at the same time by ingesting junk. Furthermore, since every physical activity has a caloric value, obesity can be effectively countered when physical activity *and* diet work together. Lifetime fitness becomes particularly valuable after weight reduction in order to *maintain* an ideal weight.

The recreational athlete or fitness person should not only have a good knowledge of food preparation but should also be his/her own nutritionist. A simple understanding of food composition and caloric value is required, if for no other reason than to counter the excessive food faddism that is characteristic of our society—and sports in particular. While faddism among ordinary eaters is bad enough, among committed exercisers it can be really dangerous. As we mentioned, erroneous beliefs at the team training tables and bizarre diets for marathoners have found their way into the public consciousness. The technique of glycogen loading, for instance, which was designed in a research laboratory in Sweden for long-term, high-endurance sports, has become the basis for an athletic eating cult here. The "running on nothing" people even advertise their habits on their T-shirts.

While glycogen repletion (or loading) is perhaps the one scientifically based diet deserving mention, it is important to understand that its application is almost entirely to very long duration, high-intensity activities like marathons or fifty-mile cross-country ski races. The average person gains nothing from this form of dietary manipulation. Nonetheless, it does help us to understand a bit more about the physiology and biochemistry of muscle contraction.

In a resting muscle, the glycogen content is usually found to be about 1.5 grams/100 grams of muscle tissue. A high-carbohydrate diet can increase muscle glycogen to about 2.5 g/100 g muscle. However, if one exercises to exhaustion (thus depleting the muscle glycogen stores) and then consumes a high-carbohydrate diet, muscle glycogen can be raised to a little over 3.0 g/100 g muscle. Yet higher levels—4 or 5 g/100 g muscle—can be achieved by exercising to exhaustion, avoiding carbohydrates for three days (eating high amounts of fat and protein), then ingesting a high carbohydrate diet for another three days. This is the diet now favored by many marathoners and cross-country ski competitors, but a notable drawback is that for every gram of glycogen stored, almost three grams of water are also stored, thus adding weight. The increase could be useful, of course, in hot weather, since the evaporation of this water aids in temperature regulation. Generally, however, the technique is most useful in those activities in which the participant might otherwise fail in the last hour or so of the competition. For a marathoner, the exhaustion that could occur in his/her final third of the race might be prevented. Cross-country skiers have been able to maintain glycogen levels sufficient for high speed through a fourth grueling hour, when, without glycogen repletion, three hours might have been their ultimate limit.

But all of this means nothing to a person whose maximum limit of exertion is pushing a pen or standing on an escalator, and little more to someone who plays tennis several times a week. It is, however, important physiologic knowledge. Of course, glycogen loading provides no guarantee of winning a marathon, especially against Bill Rodgers, who defies all nutritional truths by living on a diet of junk food, the composition of which would drive most dietitians into a frenzy of self-doubt and despair.

As you can see, if your aim is to exercise for an hour or less, daily, or somewhat less often, you should have plenty of stored energy to equip you for this amount of exertion. Dietary tinkering is unnecessary; in fact, some nutritionists argue that the frequent use of glycogen loading and other techniques may have harmful effects if carried on for months or years.

Of more important practical value is the advice that you should avoid exercising right after eating. Certainly a heavy meal is a detriment, since aside from the extra weight in your stomach the food causes the gastrointestinal system to demand extra blood, which might otherwise be needed for muscle work. In addition, your digestion may function poorly; there may even be a little regurgitation of food into the esophagus and throat. A meal taken before exercise should be light and easily digested. (You'll soon know what kinds of foods can be tolerated from your experience.) Musical and stage performers, as well as professional athletes, are familiar with this principle. In addition, candy and other sources of sugar are not only unhelpful but have been shown to severely impair performance when eaten just before you exercise.

Sugar is used *during* endurance events and (in the form of sweetened solutions) in races, but if the sugar solution is too heavy, it will tend to remain in the stomach, sometimes leading to abdominal cramps. Most well-run long-distance races have adopted a policy of fluid replacement, consistent with the climate and other conditions surrounding the race, by having "refilling stations" at regular intervals along the race route.

Dehydration can be severe in racing, and since sweat has less salt than the body's internal fluids, the body is usually water-poor, not salt-poor, during exercise of long duration. This fact makes it inadvisable to take salt replacement except under extreme conditions, such as prolonged—a week or more—exposure to hot and dry climates. The replacement of salt and other minerals by the use of prepared solutions (one of the "-ades") is controversial. Since Americans tend to use large amounts of salt in their daily diets, salt replacement is usually not only unnecessary but potentially harmful unless accompanied by adequate water intake. Thus, the athlete's proper replacement is plain water, at least in the first stages of a long run. Later, a diluted sugar solution is advised. If an electrolyte solution is offered, it should be diluted to half strength with an equal amount of water, since most "-ades" contain too concentrated a solution of salt, potassium, and sugar.

It is difficult to have a good diet when your intake is less than 2000 calories per day. (Diets of 2000 to 2500 calories, if they are properly balanced, can insure that you receive enough iron and other minerals.) This is why people who are on intermittent weight-reduction diets are often poorly nourished. The needed supplemental vitamins and iron are not found in sufficient quantity in these near-starvation regimens.

Nutritional information is both fascinating and confusing to most people, and the massive promotion of diets promising fast weight loss is testimony to our belief in magic formulas. A more realistic way to approach the weight problem is to consider 2000 calories per day as a good maintenance diet for most people, provided 2000 calories are burned off. If 2500 calories can be burned (you get a gift of about 1500 calories burned daily just from sitting around and breathing), that leaves you with a deficit of 500 calories a day, or 3500 calories a week, which equals one pound per week. At this level of intake, moreover, your diet can be nutritious if you've paid attention to its balance, as outlined in the dietary goals.

What is an ideal weight? That's one of the most vexing questions a physician must consider. Not only are most of the height-to-weight tables out of date, but they fail to take into account a number of other factors, such as body build. Also, an improvement in fitness leads to a gain in muscle mass, which of course adds weight, even if fat decreases. For that reason, skin-fold measurements are useful. A rough way to do this, suggested by the well-known nutrition expert Dr. Jean Mayer, is to pinch yourself wherever there's a lot of extra fat—under your arms, for instance. If there's more than an inch between your fingers when you remove them, you're overweight. Another way to think about ideal weight (for some people but, unhappily, not for all, since some have been overweight all their lives) is to recall when you were at some ideal weight. This could be when you got married, when you were in the military (particularly in basic training), when you were active in sports, perhaps at the end of high school or college. Try to remember how well you felt at that time. Assuming illness didn't make you skinny or malnutrition wasn't part of your upbringing, heading for that weight once more makes sense. What doesn't make sense is putting on a few pounds each year. This tendency is simply a reflection of our society's increasing use of the automobile, our dependence on fattening foods, and a misguided cultural outlook that says overweight comes with aging. But if a new standard of weight and activity can be accepted, we will all gain—or perhaps we should say *benefit*—if we lose.

5. Reducing the Chance of Injury

THE ADULT recreational athlete is, unfortunately, as susceptible to athletic injury as his/her counterpart in school or professional sports—perhaps even more so—because recreational athletes often neglect general conditioning, systematic training, and proper warm-up techniques. Of course, even with optimal fitness training, injuries will occur. But the number of injuries and their severity can be dramatically reduced with proper preparation.

Recreational athletic injuries are of two sorts, depending upon whether the injury resulted from a single major trauma, as with a direct blow from an opponent or a twisting fall in which the body weight is the deforming force, or as a result of recurrent microtrauma, such as the repetitive striking of a tennis ball with a racket or the constant footfall of running. Injuries resulting from recurrent traumas to the arms or legs are classed as *overuse* syndromes, while those resulting from major trauma are simply called *traumatic injuries.* Tennis elbow, a result of the repetitive impact of a tennis ball on the racket, is one of the more commonly encountered overuse syndromes, while a fracture of the lower leg from a twisting skiing fall is a traumatic injury.

GENERAL PREVENTIVE MEASURES

When attempting to prevent or lessen the severity of sports injuries, at least four things should be kept in mind. These include appropriate matching of participant to sport; specific training and conditioning; modification, if necessary, of the rules of the game and playing conditions; and appropriate protective equipment.

Matching of yourself to a sport is basic to injury prevention and deserves careful consideration if you are planning to engage in life sports for fitness and pleasure. While enjoyment of sports or fitness activities is important, certain people are nonetheless constitutionally ill matched to certain sports. Choosing the proper sport to begin with may be the best means of preventing problems. For example, the current running boom has swept up many people who, because of limited flexibility in their hips, or foot abnormalities, are unable to run distances without experiencing leg problems. These injury-ridden runners could save themselves significant problems by electing swimming or cycling as a life sport.

Prevention of injury by proper conditioning and training, though infinitely reasonable, has only recently been generally proven effective. Curiously, for years, conditioning, though acknowledged as essential to athletic achievement, has as often been indicated as a cause of injury rather than as a way to prevent it. At the turn of the century the enlarged "athlete's heart" of the collegiate oarsman was felt to be the result of excessive athletic activity and a direct contributor to a shorter life. We now know that this enlargement of the heart is actually a healthy response of the body to endurance training. Similarly, systematic weight training, it was said, was sure to make an athlete "muscle-bound" and was scrupulously avoided in such high-muscle-demand sports as gymnastics and dance. But it has now been well demonstrated that proper training and conditioning specifically developed for each sport not only increases the effectiveness of athletic participation but noticeably decreases the risk of injury. In both traumatic injury and overuse syndromes, a systematic muscle strengthening and flexibility program that overcomes muscle imbalances provides important protection. The emphasis must be on proper training techniques, however, since in a significant percentage of leg overuse syndromes we know that too rapid a rate of training progression can itself be a cause of injury.

Attention to game rules and playing conditions is important in decreasing the rate of severity of injury. For example, recreational hockey for adults often features a "no check" rule. Eliminating sliding into base in recreational baseball and "spiking" in recreational volleyball are other rule changes that can decrease the risk of injury.

We Americans have been considered overdependent on equipment, and the recreational athlete sometimes seems to be more interested in the latest clothes than in the sport itself. However, proper equipment does have a genuine role in injury prevention. Fortunately, most sports equipment stores are now prepared to give reasonable advice, and the sports physician or athletic trainer is another source of information.

Finally, and perhaps most important, your attitude can be instrumental in avoiding injury. Setting realistic objectives for a given sport or training is vital to avoid excessive, potentially harmful activity. Close attention should be paid to the signals of pain, overfatigue, or weakness.

FIRST AID

If injury does occur, the initial care given to a person can be absolutely crucial in reducing the extent of injury and the period of disability. The first few minutes may be the most important. For musculotendinous or extremity injuries, the steps taken to minimize further injury can be remembered by the initials I.C.E., which stand for immobilization, compression, and elevation and remind you of the need for cold applications, especially *ice*, if available.

Immobilization of an injured extremity decreases the possibility of further injury to adjacent structures and aids the mechanisms of the body that work to close off ruptured blood vessels and limit the extent of bleeding. Initial immobilization also allows the body to speed up its primary healing process of removing excess fluids and swelling from an area of injury.

Gentle compression dressings such as elastic bandages or gauze applied to an injury initially help to decrease bleeding and swelling. These dressings must never be so tightly applied as to obstruct blood flow or cause swelling below the injury. Open wounds are also best treated with direct compression applied to the wound. The application of tourniquets to an injured extremity with an open wound is usually frowned on and can be dangerous.

Early elevation of an extremity is the third step that helps to limit initial injury and decrease swelling. It is essential that the injured leg or arm be elevated above the level of the heart. Sitting in a chair with a sprained ankle on a footstool is not enough.

Finally, cooling of the injured extremity with ice packs or cold compresses also helps limit initial injury and swelling and provides pain relief. *Intermittent cooling* has proven most effective. Application of cold for five to ten minutes, followed by five to ten minutes of compression is recommended. A good combination of icing and compression can be obtained by the use of an elastic bandage that has been soaked in ice water prior to its application. We do not recommend the use of chemical coolants because the duration of their cooling effect is generally short and instances of actual burn to the skin from leaking coolant have been reported.

These general measures should be used for the first twenty-four to forty-eight hours after an injury. While specific exercises or heat may be helpful further down the line in restoring strength and function after a sports injury, their premature use may actually be harmful in certain instances.

COMMON SPORTS INJURIES

While the type and severity of injuries to the body is infinite, understanding the nature of an injury can be simplified by determining, if possible, the specific structures injured. The most common body structures injured in sports include the bones, muscle/tendon units, ligaments, cartilage, fascia, bursae, and skin.

Bones

If significant amounts of force are applied to a given bone, either as a result of a single impact, or multiple impacts, the bone can crack through. Occasionally, this question "Was it a break or a fracture?" is heard on the athletic field. They are synonymous. In a displaced bony fracture, repositioning of the bone fragments may be required, with maintenance of this repositioning by external or internal pins or plate fixation until the bone heals. This is, of course, a surgical procedure.

A stress fracture can result from repetitive activity, such as throwing or running. It is often experienced as pain alone, although swelling may be evident later. Frequently, initial X-rays of the painful bones do not show fracture, and the injury may be misdiagnosed as a tendinitis or fasciitis. Many cases of "shin splints" are in actuality stress fractures. If the arm or leg is protected early and treated by rest, complete healing results. But the best treatment of stress fracture is its prevention. Most stress fractures are the result of inappropriate training techniques with too much recurrent training over too short a period of time. Minor problems of the bones or joints, muscle imbalances, and improper footwear or running surfaces can also play a role in lower leg stress fractures. If an athlete neglects or ignores an injury by "running through pain," or if the pain warning is masked by cortisone injections or antiinflammatory medications, the stress fracture can become a complete fracture with displacement.

Muscles

Muscles have sometimes been likened to motorized rubber bands. They are the structures of the body responsible for all motion, since they can shorten themselves and exert force across the joints. They are also elastic and can be stretched to various lengths and still retain the ability to suddenly contract and exert force. Certain sports will emphasize the strength characteristic of muscles, while others will primarily demand flexibility from the muscles and their extensions, the tendons.

Injury, in a ballet dancer or weightlifter, can result from either inadequate strength or flexibility of a given muscle group.

If a muscle is exposed to excessive force a tear can occur. Such injuries are properly called muscle strain and include the playing field diagnoses of "muscle pull" and "charley horse."

Studies of muscle strains in a variety of sports give clues to their prevention. These often occur early in the season, and in players who are "tight" and have not warmed up properly. In addition, athletes who have not followed a balanced training program and have concentrated on strengthening one set of muscles without also strengthening the opposite ones are likely to strain the weaker muscle set. For example, sprinters or hurdlers who work primarily on strengthening the muscle in the front of the thigh without also strengthening (and stretching) the hamstring muscles in the back of the thigh are particularly subject to "pulled" hamstrings. Proper warm-up and a balanced strengthening and stretching program for "high demand muscles" in a given sport are the best ways to prevent muscle strain.

While muscle strains are often classed as "nuisance" injuries, they can cause significant disability and may even require hospitalization or extended crutch support if a major muscle is torn. Extended periods of exercise are frequently required to restore strength and flexibility to these injured muscles. Tears of the inner calf muscles in tennis players ("tennis leg"), tears of the hamstrings in runners, and tears of the muscles of the upper and midback in canoers and rowers suggest that participants in these sports cannot neglect proper conditioning of their muscles.

Muscles and adjacent soft tissue are also subject to contusions—localized swelling usually due to a direct blow of sufficient force to produce tissue injury and rupture blood vessels. Contusions are often referred to as "lumps," or if accompanied by bleeding, "bruises." All too often such localized injuries result from poor playing techniques or inadequate protective equipment. While generally minor in extent and degree of disability, contusions of major muscles, such as the thigh, can cause severe pain and prolonged disability. We have seen a thigh contusion in a soccer player permanently limit knee mobility and a forearm contusion in a hockey player actually threaten the blood supply to the hand because of extensive swelling.

In all contusions, early use of immobilization, compression, elevation, and icing can help to limit your disability. In severe contusions, intermittent icing may be continued for up to five to seven days following injury. While the application of heat or the use of warm whirlpools may help restore flexibility and joint motion, use of these too soon after an injury can actually cause further bleeding and prolong disability rather than shorten it. In a severe contusion, we tend to err on the side of caution and follow the five- to seven-day icing routine.

Tendons

Sometimes an acute injury or chronic overuse injury of a muscle/tendon unit can result in an injury to the tendon alone. Known as tendinitis, it causes pain and swelling and often limits the motion of an adjacent joint. This inflammation is usually the result of small tears or irritations of the actual substance of the tendon. The resultant pain and disability is due to the body's normal mechanism of healing any injury of its tissue. It causes us to stop and rest the injured element. But this pain feedback to the brain inhibits our use of the entire leg or arm involved, with a decrease in its bulk, strength, and endurance. Thus a vicious cycle can begin in which the initial muscle or structural imbalance that caused the tendinitis in the first place is further exaggerated by the inhibitory effect of the pain.

In such a situation, great care must be taken in the use of antiinflammatory drugs or cortisone injections. Though they may give temporary relief by decreasing the swelling or interrupting normal pain pathways, the primary condition usually persists. Unless specific steps are taken to alter the weakness, more serious injury may result. A good example of this is Achilles' tendinitis, or inflammation of the tendon of the heel. This painful injury is often the result of a single episode of overuse, such as a weekend bike ride. In this situation, proper initial treatment includes resting the muscle and tendon and using ice compresses and mild antiinflammatory medications such as aspirin. When the acute stages of injury have subsided, and when there is a decrease of the swelling and pain, corrective measures such as stretching of the calf muscles and strengthening of the muscles in the front of the leg should be started to improve the primary condition, which is usually a muscle imbalance about the lower leg. If, instead, cortisone is injected into the tendon and no further corrective measures are taken, the medication may mask further small tears in the tendon, which can lead to complete rupture of the heel cord.

Alternatively, repeated episodes of Achilles' tendinitis, in which activity is resumed before complete healing has occurred and in which no attempt is made to correct the primary muscle/tendon imbalance, can result in progressive scar formation to the point where surgery may be required.

Well known to many is rotator cuff tendinitis, which occurs about the shoulder and is a big problem in racquet sports. As detailed in chapter seven, this condition is most often the result of improper training, muscle weakness, and lack of flexibility about the entire shoulder joint. It is most properly corrected, over the long term, by the right kind of stretching and strengthening exercises and the practice of slow, progressive training techniques.

Joints

As a result of the many different structures and tissues making up or spanning a given joint—including ligaments, cartilage, nerves, blood vessels, and tendons—determination of the structures responsible for pain, stiffness, or disability at a joint can be difficult.

For example, "tennis elbow" is actually a tendinitis of the muscles on the back of the arm at the elbow; "runner's knee" is an irritation of the cartilage of the knee joint; and "football knee" is usually a loose knee resulting from injuries to the ligaments of the knee joint.

Dislocation is a complete separation and displacement of the two or more bones making up a joint. It is accompanied by significant injury to the ligaments and muscle/tendon units spanning the joint and should be considered a medical emergency. In many cases, dislocation of a major joint causes partial obstruction of the blood flow or nerve supply to the arm or leg. Treatment should be carried out as quickly as possible. Dislocations of the elbow, knee, or ankle are most serious. But dislocations of the fingers or toes, although often easily treated on the field, should also always be evaluated by a physician, since they too can result in permanent disability.

A partial displacement of the joints, usually transient in nature, is called a *subluxation.* The most common form seen in athletics is in the shoulder. We have seen that muscle imbalances or tightness can play a role in causing subluxations, or even dislocations, about joints.

Sprains

A sprain is a joint injury of the ligaments and usually results from deformation or excessive motion of the joint. Sprains are classed as first, second, or third degree depending on the extent of disruption of the ligaments and the instability of the joint. In a first-degree sprain, there is tenderness and swelling over the ligament, but the joint is stable. In a second-degree sprain, there is some instability of the joint in addition to tenderness and swelling, but the ligament is only partially separated and retains some mechanical stability. In a third-degree sprain, there is complete tearing of the ligament, usually with loss of stability of the joint on the side of the ligament ruptured.

While third-degree or complete ligament tears usually require surgical repair, first- and second-degree sprains can usually be treated by I.C.E. first-aid measures and then restored to full motion and strength by appropriate muscle strengthening and flexibility exercises. Even though, after a second-degree ligament rupture, some increased looseness of the joint may be evident, specific strengthening of the muscles and tendons spanning this joint can often more than adequately substitute for the injured ligament. As an example, second-degree ankle sprains rarely result in permanent disability if proper rehabilitation exercises, including stretching of the heel cord and strengthening of the muscle in front of the leg, are performed after the early healing stage.

Joints that are relatively stiff and lacking in flexibility appear to be particularly susceptible to sprains and, once again, the best prevention of these ligament injuries appears to be stretching and flexibility exercises that maintain full motion about the joints. Finally, sprains should never be minimized since lack of restoration of proper strength and flexibility can lead to further injury of significantly increased severity.

Back Injuries

Back ailments are now one of our major medical problems. It is estimated that one in three Americans will have major trouble with his/her back at some time. While sports participation can help strengthen the back and protect it from injury, as often as not a serious back injury resulting in three or four weeks of lost work time has been precipitated by a tennis stroke, a basketball jump, or even jogging.

The back is a complex structure of bones, ligaments, muscles, tendons, nerves, and, of course, the intervertebral discs that connect each portion of the bony spine and cushion impact to the back and spine. While a back injury may involve one or several of these structures, the most common protective mechanism of the back occurs when its muscles go into spasm and tighten up.

The best way to prevent back injury, and, in fact, the best long-term treatment following back injury, is to stretch the muscles on the back of the torso and strengthen those in front, while avoiding anything that puts excessive strain upon the back. "Lift with the legs, and not the back" is as pertinent to the playing field or the court as it is to the job. The first lesson any beginning weightlifter must learn is how to lift without putting excessive strain upon the back. While few of us will engage in competitive weightlifting, all of us must learn the techniques of back protection and how to maintain a strong and flexible back and abdomen. The back exercise program in the Appendix should be a part of the training program for every sport.

Head Injuries

While head injuries are rare in recreational sports, they can occur unexpectedly, and the results can be tragic. One of our colleagues recently found himself as a patient in the neurosurgical unit of a hospital after falling off his bicycle. While the brain is well protected from direct injury by the heavy bones of the skull on its top and sides, blows delivered to the base of the brain or the jaw can result in significant indirect injury to the brain as it bounces back and forth off the inner surface of the skull. Such brain injuries as loss of consciousness and significant change in mental function are called *concussions.* Fortunately, the results of such injuries are usually transient, although serious brain injury or even death can occur from a relatively minor trauma.

Our colleague now dons a protective helmet while cycling, and it is evident that wearing proper headgear—where there is potential for significant impact injury to the head in such sports as riding, kayaking, and hockey—is necessary. Similarly, prevention of injuries to the eyes, nose, and mouth calls for the right kind of protective equipment.

Eye Injuries

Eye injuries must always be treated with the greatest respect, particularly if there is blurring of vision or sensitivity to light and excessive tearing of the eye. The injured eye should be closed and covered with soft cotton dressing held in place with wrappings and the injured athlete should be taken immediately to an emergency facility or ophthalmologist. Certain eye injuries may be painless and can be detected only by a minimal blurring of vision in the affected eye. Despite this, immediate evaluation is recommended since delay in treatment can result in permanent damage to vision.

Recent studies have shown that the numbers and severity of injuries to the eyes can be dramatically reduced by the use of eye protective equipment in racquet sports (see chapter seven) and in any other sport where a rapidly moving projectile is used. Clearly, the benefits of proper eye protection far outweigh the relatively minor inconvenience of protective eyeglasses or goggles.

Mouth Injuries

Injuries to the mouth and teeth, while somewhat unusual, can occur in a great variety of sports. Whether the result of a blow from an opponent's racquet or elbow, or a stumbling fall while jogging, certain basic principles of first aid should be known.

If a tooth has been knocked out, it should be retrieved and both the tooth and mouth washed out with plain water to remove particles of tooth, dirt, gravel, and loose, injured tissue. The tooth should then be replaced in the socket and the injured athlete taken immediately to a dentist or oral surgeon.

If, after a mouth injury, the teeth are all in place but there is some bleeding detectable about the gums, or if there is increased sensitivity to touch in one or more of the teeth, there may be injury to the tooth or its socket. Once again, further evaluation is important. Closely fitted mouthguards, usually made for the upper teeth alone, can noticeably reduce teeth and mouth injury. These protective devices are recommended in basketball, rugby, soccer, and hockey and in any sport situation where blows about the jaw or mouth are possible.

Thermal Injury

Problems caused by weather can be anything from a small annoyance to a life-threatening disaster. Heat, cold, and wind are factors in our daily lives, though for the most part we can insulate ourselves against extremes. The same is not true, say, for a lightly clothed runner who, after running several miles in wet, cold weather, will be susceptible to one kind of cold injury. This is *hypothermia*—the lowering of the body's temperature to dangerous levels. On the other hand, if the weather is hot and humid, the same person could be felled by heat exhaustion or heat stroke. In some seasons, when weather changes are frequent, these extremes can occur within days of each other.

Most thermal injury is preventable, given common sense and a little forethought. While in large-scale athletic events the planners will often have provisions to counteract thermal injury and to provide emergency medical care, every athlete should know the basics of prevention and treatment of thermal injury.

The resistance of an athlete to thermal injury—either heat or cold—can be increased by a period of exposure and training in that environment. Heat acclimatization calls for a progressive exercise program done in the heat for a period of five to eight days. Simply resting in the heat will not result in acclimatization. The mechanism of this acclimatization is primarily "salt saving." The body decreases the salt it secretes in the urine and sweat, despite losses of up to fifteen pounds of body weight as water.

Cold acclimatization takes much longer to acquire—on the order of three to four weeks—and amounts to selective changes in the blood flow to the trunk and extremities. Here the body maintains the temperature of its central core while allowing the temperature of the extremities to decrease.

With either heat or cold exposure, proper acclimatization is the first step in the prevention of injury.

There are three major types of heat injury: heat cramps, heat exhaustion, and heat stroke. The first, heat cramps, is unlikely to occur in recreational sports, while the other two are more common problems. The underlying principle in preventing and treating heat exhaustion and heat stroke is: *replace water.*

Heat exhaustion actually comes in two versions, that caused by predominant water loss and that caused by predominant salt loss, both in unacclimatized persons. If water is not replaced—some experts say it should be in *excess* of need—or if the person affected can't express a need for water because he/she is unconscious or confused, then heat exhaustion results, its symptoms and signs being thirst, agitation, weakness, fatigue, anxiety, and impaired judgment. When not treated, mental and neurological dysfunctions will occur and the condition can progress to heat stroke. The most obvious outward sign is an elevated temperature.

For heat exhaustion, the person should be put in a cool place. Usually recovery is fairly rapid. Water replacement is essential.

Heat stroke (heat hyperpyrexia, sunstroke) is most likely to occur in people with some chronic illness or deficiency of the sweating mechanism. Its occasional occurrence in a runner or other athletic participant is more likely to happen if there are other problems such as a recent viral infection, fever, or a potassium deficiency, which can occur in diarrhea.

In general, a healthy individual is likely to suffer heat stroke in any situation where the body's ability to get rid of excess heat is impaired. In the inexperienced athlete who doesn't know how to pace an activity—young, highly competitive, and overenthusiastic persons, mostly—heat stroke is a danger, particularly in humid climates, where evaporation is poor.

There is a myth that water should be withheld from some competitors; this is wrong. The person suffering heat stroke usually stops sweating at a certain point. Temperature rises to dangerously high levels. He/she may lose consciousness, often suddenly. If the person is awake, he/she may have headache, dizziness, and mental confusion. Shock—a sudden and disastrous drop in blood pressure—may occur. Heat stroke is a true emergency.

First aid consists of taking the person to a cool place, undressing him/her, and assisting evaporation by applying water, iced if possible. Fanning and massage can be used initially if ice water is not available. Another method of treating heat stroke is to apply tepid water and to blow air across the body with fans, evaporating the water and thereby cooling the body. Some would argue that ice water can so constrict peripheral blood vessels that cooling is not as efficiently produced as it is with tepid water. In a hospital, cooling baths or cooling blankets are used and will save most of those affected by heat stroke. Since there are possible circulatory and kidney problems, patients with heat stroke must be hospitalized and watched for several days to insure against complications.

It is important to understand that heat stroke is a severe disturbance that can be fatal. Cooling (to levels below 102° F. or 38.9° C.) and immediate transfer to a hospital are essential. In the absence of good first-aid treatment, the chance of death or permanent impairment is high.

Preparation for sports participation in the heat—by acclimatization if possible—is the first step in prevention. If the athlete has reason to doubt his/her acclimatization, as on an unseasonably warm, humid day in early spring, prolonged activity should be avoided. In addition, even with the acclimatized athlete, regular water intake should be continued—at least a glass of water every fifteen to twenty minutes. Recent studies have shown that various beverage mixes containing salt or sugar, and billed as "sports beverages," actually are less effective than water alone in preventing heat injury, and, if used for refreshment during sports, should be diluted two to three times with water.

Cold Injury

Like their heat-associated counterparts, injuries at the cold extreme can be minor or major, the latter possibly being fatal. The major problems for persons who perform outdoors during cold weather are frost-nips, frostbite, and hypothermia.

Frost-nips and frostbite are simply the first stages of cold injury. In all cold injury, the blood vessels in the exposed area react by constricting, thus shunting blood away from the skin and to the internal organs. This is a way of preserving the functions of the organs themselves—by keeping the body's core temperature at a normal level. What blood there is in chilled skin will itself be chilled and, upon its return to the body's interior, will affect organs adversely. As the blood is shunted away from the skin, the skin becomes more vulnerable to cold injury. Ultimately, the body may actually sacrifice a cold-injured portion of an arm or leg in order to preserve the functioning of the brain, kidneys, heart, and other vital organs.

Modern treatment of these disorders takes into account the body's own "logic" in dealing with the injury.

The most important variable in any cold injury is the wind-chill factor. If the temperature is 30° F., being outdoors on a windless day in proper clothing isn't unsafe or uncomfortable. However, at the same temperature, plus a wind of 25 mph, the wind-chill factor is 0°. In other words, your thermometer gives you only part of the story. The real temperature for your body's purposes can be far lower, and you must protect yourself accordingly.

Frost-nips (easily treated) are suddenly occurring white spots on exposed areas or on covered fingers and toes. It is important to avoid hand rubbing of such injury—particularly with snow. As one expert has commented, that's a lot like sticking a badly burned arm in a hot oven. The treatment is gentle massage by a warm hand, or cupping the hands and blowing into them, thus rechanneling the breath toward the

WIND CHILL CHART*

Wind Speed (MPH) — Temperature (Thermometer Reading, Fahrenheit)

Wind Speed (MPH)	50	40	30	20	10	0	-10	-20	-30	-40	-50
	Equivalent Temperature										
5	48	37	27	16	6	-5	-15	-26	-36	-47	-57
10	40	28	16	4	-9	-24	-33	-46	-58	-70	-83
15	36	22	9	-5	-18	-32	-45	-58	-72	-85	-99
20	32	18	4	-10	-25	-39	-53	-67	-82	-96	-110
25	30	16	0	-15	-29	-44	-59	-74	-88	-104	-118
30	28	13	-2	-18	-33	-48	-63	-79	-94	-109	-125
35	27	11	-4	-21	-35	-51	-67	-82	-98	-113	-129
40	26	10	-6	-21	-37	-53	-69	-85	-100	-115	-132

Wind speeds greater than forty miles per hour have little additional effect.

*From James A. Wilkerson, M.D., ed., *Medicine for Mountaineering* (Seattle, Washington: The Mountaineers, 1975), p. 155.

face; or, if necessary, putting the feet or hands in someone's armpit. Usually that's all that's necessary. But if untreated, frost damage to the skin can progress to frostbite. In this connection, it is important to remember that refreezing is to be avoided at all costs.

Frostbite is a serious and potentially disfiguring injury. Feet and hands are particularly vulnerable, and there seems to be more likelihood of such injury under conditions of panic (when increased perspiration may result and enhance cold transmission through clothing) or illness, exhaustion, or poor nutritional status.

Often the first sign that frost-nip is becoming frostbite is a pleasant sensation of absence of pain or discomfort. Cold toes that become more comfortable during severe cold circumstances are announcing that they have become frozen, their normal pain-relaying systems now closed down along with their blood supply. At this stage, which is still early enough to treat on the trail, the affected part can be removed from boots or mitts, and put against someone's body, on the belly, for instance.

It is important to remember that wet clothing reduces the insulating effect of fabric many times over. Hiking in such gear is not only uncomfortable but downright foolish. If the injury is at the frost-nip stage as described here, the clothing must be dried out or a substitute set of gear put on before proceeding.

The serious effects of frostbite—loss of toes or fingers, for instance—are often the result of too vigorous treatment. As mentioned, hard rubbing of the affected part or massaging it with snow must be avoided at all costs. Furthermore, it is extremely dangerous to thaw out an affected part and then allow it to refreeze. It is far better to allow the frostbitten part to stay frozen until you reach a warm environment, where thawing can take place gradually and safely and medical attention can be given. A person whose feet are frozen is actually capable of hiking out of an area, while one whose feet have been thawed will require assistance, not always an easy task under the circumstances. Records show that the recovery rate is much greater for those who follow this advice, compared with those whose limbs were treated and then allowed to refreeze.

Treatment of frostbitten extremities takes great patience and the utmost avoidance of radical measures. Nature's way of healing these areas is slow but often surprisingly complete. A number of excellent manuals covering all aspects of frostbite exist and should be familiar to anyone hiking in or otherwise experiencing extremes of cold for any period of time.

Hypothermia, on the other hand, is a condition capable of killing humans at temperatures that might be considered, at the worst, mild. Hikers have experienced hypothermia in the summer as well as the winter. The problem—loss of the heat at the body's core—is caused by the rapid removal of heat from the skin, faster than it can be replaced by the body's own heat-producing processes.

When clothing is inadequate for the climate, when conditioning is lacking, or when injury makes exercise impossible, hypothermia may strike. Shivering will be the first sign of trouble, but later shivering will lessen as the muscles become rigid and mental confusion begins. This confusion accounts for the frequent occurrence, under arctic or severe mountain conditions, of bizarre behavior in badly chilled persons—often a prelude to wandering off from camp or inability to follow group efforts. Eventually, death may occur from the effect of cold upon those parts of the brain that control heart and lung functions.

With hypothermia, rapid rewarming of the body is to be avoided, unless one is prepared to resuscitate, since rewarming forces the cooled blood in the skin and peripheral parts of the body to suddenly find its way into the heart and lungs, making cardiac arrest possible. Cardiopulmonary resuscitation may become necessary. Slow and gradual rewarming is best.

Heat is lost from the body by four avenues: *conduction* (through direct contact with cooler surfaces such as the ground or rocks), *radiation* (to cooler areas near or far away, such as walls, rocks, or the atmosphere, irrespective of the temperature of the air nearby), *convection* (the setting up of air currents at the body's surface because of the relatively warmer air there), and *evaporation* (sweating—which requires that extra heat be produced by the body).

There are several ways to prevent heat loss. Shivering is one of the body's principal defenses against cold. It is a highly efficient mechanism, though appropriate only for moderate cold. The heat produced is roughly equivalent to that produced during slow running. Another of the body's defenses is constriction of the blood vessels of the skin—the same mechanism that leads to frostbite, of course. Less heat is thereby lost from the body's core, since the skin now acts as an insulator and the remaining heat can be used by the relatively smaller group of vital organs whose functions must be preserved at all cost.

Finally, clothing can reduce or promote heat loss. If wet, its insulating properties are greatly impaired, but if dry and layered, with air between, its insulating properties are enhanced. Since about half of your body's heat is lost through the scalp, a hat is more than a head decoration—it's an efficient insulator.

Lightning Injury

Lightning tends to seek out any prominent object in an area. A soccer player on a field or a hiker on an exposed ridge is particularly vulnerable. The most important thing to understand about a person who has been struck by lightning is that his/her life can probably be saved by cardiopulmonary resuscitation.

Unfortunately, there is a kind of fatalistic attitude about lightning strikes—part of our mythic heritage—that seems to paralyze bystanders. People who would readily assist a person who has collapsed in the street tend to avoid the lightning victim. Of course, there is also the practical danger of being struck oneself and the natural tendency is to seek a safe place. If help can be given, though, it may well prove to be lifesaving.

The injury from lightning is an electrical disturbance of the heart or the respiratory center in the brain. Maintenance of an airway, mouth-to-mouth breathing, and closed-chest cardiac massage are the tools for saving the victim's life. Since time is limited, assistance must be given immediately. Somewhere between 150 and 300 persons die annually in the United States because of lightning strikes; most of them could have been resuscitated if assistance had been given.

The burns that occur at the point of entry and exit of the electrical current can be treated like any other burn and will generally heal without any complications.

Most important, weather and outdoor conditions must be treated with respect. Humans have adapted to the vagaries of their habitat, but not always perfectly, and the "human element"—which usually means judgment, or lack of it—often operates in such a way as to promote foolish chance-taking. Respect for conditions rather than heroics is the rule.

II
LIFE SPORTS

The muscular requirements of each life sport differ in some important ways. In addition, each physical activity described in the following chapters has specific training needs and specific strengthening effects upon the body and is subject to specific injuries. Our desire is to illustrate in the simplest manner the attributes of each of a number of sports that adults might enjoy and use as a means of becoming and staying fit.

This is by no means a complete list; in certain respects, it represents our biases. Some readers may be disappointed that a favorite sport has been omitted. To them, we can say only that our choices represent a reasonable, but not complete, cross section of activities available to people, each of which is capable of contributing positively to health.

For each sport, we have two sets of diagrams. Opening each chapter are drawings of active people actively engaged in the sports described in the chapter. The solid circles indicate the muscles that need to be strengthened by the exercises suggested in the Appendix and the broken-line circles indicate the muscles that need to be stretched. Immediately following these drawings are two charts in which the parts of the body that need to be stretched or strengthened for the sport are indicated by bullets. (As we have said earlier, stretching exercises increase flexibility, while strengthening workouts improve endurance.) In addition, each sports chapter describes the strengthening effect of the sport itself; in other words, what muscles does it affect favorably?

Energy consumption is included whenever it can be calculated. In the Appendix we provide detailed descriptions and illustrations of all the stretching and strengthening exercises.

Our hope is that the chapters in part two will lead you to a safe and flexible program that does not commit you to any one sport, but allows you to change and flow with the season with your personal likes and dislikes and with the availability of facilities.

For most sports, a general warm-up, in addition to specific stretching and strengthening exercises, is desirable. In many cases, all this means is that you should perform the sport (running, cycling) at a slow pace, perhaps two or three times around a given course, and then do a few jumping jacks and some trunk rolls. By working up a light sweat, you will increase the circulation to those muscles that will be more active later and prepare them for heavier use. Warm-ups should require no more than five or ten minutes, although in cold weather the requirement might be longer. Many of the stretching exercises listed in the sports chapters can be used as warm-ups as well.

It is through sports that you can become fit for sports. Some overlap, particularly in the cardiovascular area, exists between sports, even though each activity has its own specific training needs. By following the general conditioning principles described earlier, and by observing the training rules for each of the sports about to be described, you should develop a stronger and more energetic body.

Finally, remember that fun *is the most important ingredient!*

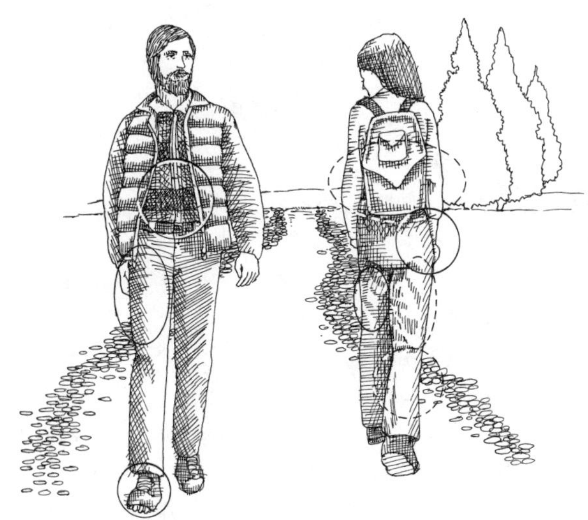

6. Walking, Hiking, Running, Orienteering

Energy Consumption:

Slow walking or strolling at 1 mile/hr.	135 cals./hr.
Level walking at 2 miles/hr.	200 cals./hr.
Slightly brisk pace of 3 miles/hr.	270 cals./hr.
Brisk walking at 3.5 miles/hr.	330 cals./hr.
Faster yet at 4 miles/hr.	400 cals./hr.
Rapid walking at 5 miles/hr.	450 cals./hr.
Jogging at 5 miles/hr. (slow jog)	550 cals./hr.
Running at 5.5 miles/hr.	630 cals./hr.
Running at 7 miles/hr.	750 cals./hr.

Strengthening Effect: calf musculature (the thighs, contrary to popular belief, are not strengthened).

Stretching exercises:

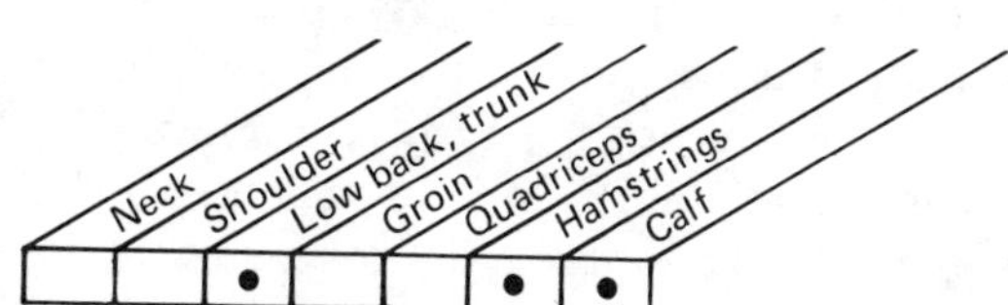

Neck	Shoulder	Low back, trunk	Groin	Quadriceps	Hamstrings	Calf
		•			•	•

Strengthening exercises:

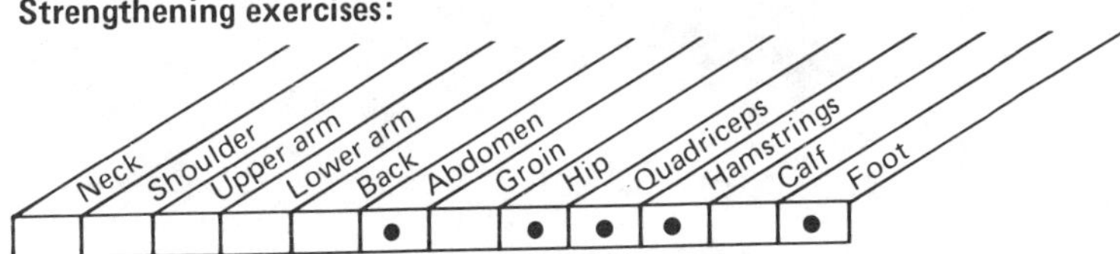

RUNNING—or jogging, the peculiarly American version of the sport—became the fastest-growing sport of the 1970s. Its immense popularity, in addition to its low start-up costs, has caused it to overshadow most of the other leg-powered activities, if not all other physical outlets. Some of our patients sometimes shamefacedly admit that they don't jog, as if that were an admission of guilt. Our answer is that there are plenty of other things to do, including walking.

Those familiar with the history of sports will wonder whether jogging is yet another of those crazes that will burn out, or transform itself on the other hand into a purely competitive sport, offsetting the potential cardiovascular benefits of a stronger heart and high calorie utilization now enjoyed by recreational joggers. There are signs of compulsiveness among many runners, and competition now exists at the local level in the form of "fun runs." Competition rules at that level and on up through the level of the marathon.

Nonetheless, running evokes some of the most basic patterns of human response, frees people from the usual constraints of a daily life in a car or at a desk, and is a superb conditioner.

Competition isn't necessary to enjoy its many benefits, and our intention is not to add another rhapsody to the already bloated literature. Instead, we will call attention to the requirements for conditioning as well as the potential for musculoskeletal damage—which is considerable—and we will try to put the whole field of "leg-sports" into a more balanced perspective.

WALKING

The first and most important of leg sports is walking. The history of walking is long and the sport has often been praised in literature. Many British and American writers of the nineteenth century wrote essays on walking, or claimed to have been inspired by walking. The English novelist George Meredith was probably the champion literary walker of his time and (in common with other contemporary writers) celebrated it as a way of gaining health and overcoming depression (or, as the state was then known, melancholia). Emerson's view was that few are born good walkers; he thought it desirable to publish an "Art of Walking, with Easy Lessons for Beginners." A professional walker, Emerson said, would arrive at that state by persisting from year to year, obtaining "at least an intimacy with the country, and know all the good points within ten miles, with the reasons for visiting each, know the lakes, the hills, where grapes, berries and nuts, where the rare plants are; where the best botanic ground; and where the noblest landscapes are seen."

Our society, with a higher value on highways for automobiles than footpaths for people, places obstacles in our way when we wish to walk. The concept of private property in this country severely limits our access to places for walking. In Scandinavia, where all land is open for walking, hiking, skiing, running, and other activities, the concept of private property is vastly different from that in North America. You might own land or a vacation place, but you can't prohibit someone from using your property, so long as he/she doesn't disturb your peace or damage your belongings or land. This principle—Everyman's Right, it is called—goes back to the custom, in the Middle Ages, of berry picking in the woods. In other words, the berries, and thus the woods, belong to everyone. That simple idea makes available to the public a vast network of hiking and walking trails. As a result, the Scandinavian people tend to look to the out-of-doors for their recreation and, at the same time, place a high value on conservation of their natural resources.

When robust Victorians talked about walking, they included

what we think of as hiking. Climbing a height of land became part of the normal activity of many people in the nineteenth century, either in solitary fashion or in the company of fellow members of a walking club. The mountaineering tradition, so much a part of the "manly" attitudes of the British of the time, probably grew out of these walking expeditions.

Since the areas for walking are so accessible, it makes sense to walk whenever we can. The number of calories burned is governed by the distance covered, not the speed of movement, so walking is a very efficient alternative to other sports and should be high on one's list of aerobic sports. Walking up stairs, walking to church, walking to the store, walking the dog are all good conditioners and can be inserted into your daily routine on a regular basis. As we have mentioned, a significant number of calories can be burned off in such a manner, aiding weight control.

It is not widely known that the surface you walk on affects the amount of energy used. A smooth concrete or asphalt surface will require about three quarters of the energy needed to walk across a plowed field. Walking up stairs is twice as energy-consuming as walking on the level, though going down requires very little, about one third of that needed for going up. As in many activities, a heavier person burns off more calories than a thinner one.

HIKING

Hiking is a step removed from walking, and preparation for this activity should ideally be started several weeks before a hike. This can consist of stair-climbing and should include quadriceps strengthening, since the downhill component of hiking places great strain upon the front of the thigh. Poor development there can easily lead to knee problems, with pain and swelling the occasional result. Training includes walking, at least a half hour a day, preferably longer. Boring as it might be, racing up and down stadium steps is an excellent way to prepare.

Clothing is of great importance in hiking. Boots must be sturdy, providing support for the ankle, and their soles should be of Vibram or similar hard rubber with treads. While there are a large number of specialized items of footwear and clothing for various types of mountain hiking, the most important step for a novice hiker is to get properly fitting boots. Footwear that fits poorly can cause agonizing pain in the feet or toes on an extended hike. Two pairs of socks are usually worn, a thinner cotton one first, a wool sock outside. The purpose of this is to draw moisture away from the feet. Boots and socks must not fit too tightly, or circulation will be compromised. The rest of your clothing must be adapted to the climate and possible sudden changes in temperature and wind conditions. Hiking in the mountains can expose people to unpredictable weather, and a warm spring day at the bottom can turn into a raging winter storm at the top of a mountain. You must carry enough layers of clothing to prevent hypothermia, though some of them might have to be carried in a knapsack on warm days.

RUNNING

While amateur running, unlike hiking, requires no training period, it should be taken up gradually—starting with walking and then moving to walking and jogging alternately. A reasonable program for any beginner might be a "five and ten" schedule: five minutes of walking separated by ten of jogging. This is really a form of interval training and, if pulse rates or the "talk test" are used as guides, will result in an increased aerobic capacity within a period of six weeks to three months. At this point, jogging could be the principal outlet, but walking should nonetheless be done at every opportunity during the rest of the day. Adequate levels of aerobic fitness, for most people, can be maintained by running no less than three times a week, for about thirty minutes each time. The beginning runner, though, must use a program of five to ten minutes every other day at first, gradually, over the ensuing weeks, lengthening his/her time.

Unlike swimming or cycling, running causes a striking action of the feet and legs with each step. This recurrent microtrauma can even break bones. Thus, a walking program prior to more active exercise makes sense, for it gives the bones and muscles time to prepare: the bones can remodel themselves and become stronger and the muscles stretch and strengthen.

A relaxed feeling while jogging and proper warm-up are necessary. Your head should be up and your body upright. Your arms should be bent so that the forearms are parallel to the ground and held slightly away from the body. Any relaxation procedure (deep breathing, meditation, shaking yourself loose) is good preparation.

Keep jogging clothing simple; in warm weather, light shorts and a porous shirt are fine. Men will want to have scrotal support of some sort for comfort; women may wish not to wear a bra. (In our discussion of the female athlete we cited a survey taken of women on this subject, pointing out that it is really a matter of personal like and dislike. There is no evidence that running bra-less causes any harm to the support structures of the female breast.) Under no circumstances should rubberized or sweat-retaining materials be worn. When we lose weight by sweating, all we are losing is water, which is gained back almost immediately. Its loss has no relevance to weight reduction. Besides, the heat-retaining effort may cause hyperthermic states like heat exhaustion. In colder weather a hat is important, since about half the body's heat loss is through the scalp.

There is a great mystique about running shoes today, but you can go to a shop specializing in running shoes and equipment in almost all good-sized cities and find decent equipment for your feet. The running magazines print reviews of shoes, and companies produce advertisements with specifications listed that make the footwear resemble stereo equipment in their complexity. The main job of the running shoe is to cushion the impact of the foot against a hard surface. Since most Americans run on pavement, that's really very important. Moreover, sneakers or tennis shoes, which lack the side-to-side rigidity of running shoes (tennis players and others must make fast breaks from one side to the other, as opposed to runners, who are always running in a forward direction), are inadequate for running and their use may result in significant injury—

particularly a painful condition of the heel cord known as plantar fasciitis (inflammation of the fibrous tissues of the sole of the foot). When this occurs, you are likely to awake each morning with a burning pain under your heel; if you're lucky, it will ease up during the day. Otherwise you may find yourself in the hands of a specialist for definitive treatment.

Running has been the main sport responsible for the rapid expansion of sports medicine programs. Most of the specialists in this area—orthopedists, trainers, podiatrists—formerly treated big-league athletes and professional players, with a sprinkling of other patients. Now the runners have arrived on the scene, and clinics are full of people whose feet, knees, hips, shins, and other lower extremity parts are aching, tight, swollen, or bruised. In fact, running has caused a revolution in podiatry, a specialty heretofore confined almost exclusively to paring the corns and clipping the toenails of elderly and incapacitated individuals. Not that podiatrists didn't have skills: they have always been highly trained and competent specialists in foot care. It's just that the public didn't put much value on its feet until recently. Now podiatrists are seen as vital allies in the effort to keep people running, and the public regards them with a deserved respect.

Understandably, the foot is the site of most difficulties in walking and hiking. Blisters from poorly fitting footwear are common. When they do occur, they should be protected with a dressing, not broken. The fluid present under the blister assists in healing; if the blister is broken, infection can start. Poorly broken in hiking boots are often a source of much of this trouble. Unclipped toenails can be very painful, for on a hike, as you go downhill, your long toenails will jam into the front of your boot. Needless to say, this will test your capacity for pain endurance. A similar problem occurs with runners if their shoes are too small or narrow at the tip. *Runner's toes* are hemorrhages under the toenails caused by the repeated trauma of jamming the toes against the front of the shoe. While they are colorful, they aren't dangerous, but they are a sign that you should have purchased better-fitting shoes. *Immersion foot* can be experienced by hikers. This cold injury is the result of wet, cold water in contact with the feet. Dry footgear is, of course, essential for proper hiking, so spare socks and some alternate shoes should be carried; gentle rewarming will take care of immersion foot.

If pre-hiking or pre-running stretching of the Achilles' tendon has not been sufficient to prevent tendinitis and fasciitis in the heel and heel cord, a plastic insert known as an *orthotic* may be necessary. A sports medicine specialist can be helpful here.

Knee and hip problems are common in hikers and runners. A knee that functions perfectly well under unstressful conditions may begin to act up when overuse occurs. In extreme situations, the knee can become swollen with fluid that accumulates inside the joint. Often, this is the result of inadequate training of the quadriceps muscle, which is the large muscle at the front of the thigh, or because of an imbalance between the two portions of the muscle attached to the kneecap, the *vastus medialis* and the *vastus lateralis.* Quadriceps strengthening exercises are necessary to counteract this tendency to knee strain and are relatively simple to do. They make good sense for anyone embarking on a running program. In fact, "runner's knee" is also cyclist's, cross-country skier's, skater's, and (in swimming) frog-kicker's knee. The problem—a roughening of the backside of the kneecap—is becoming quite common, as more and more people engage in physical activity.

Certainly there is a need for training before such problems start. Quadriceps exercises are shown in the Appendix. One good way to carry them out is to sit on the edge of a desk or table and raise your leg until it is fully extended, then lower it slowly. This can be done for up to ten times without additional weight on the foot. After sufficient strengthening has occurred, a weight can be added—a heavy shoe, small sandbag or a boot can serve. An office "exercise break" provides a good opportunity to carry this out.

Unusual strain and stresses placed upon the knee or ankle—twisting or shearing forces occurring as a result of falls or slips, for instance, need to be attended to immediately and may require immobilization with splints or crutches. If ice is available, it should be applied to all new areas of injury. Since in some cases a fracture of a bone may be involved, X-rays are often necessary. The extreme pain and other changes occurring in certain fractures will sometimes cause a person to go into shock, with low blood pressure, clammy skin, and a rapid pulse. The patient needs to be bundled up with warm clothes and blankets, with his/her feet placed higher than the head, and be transported to an emergency room immediately. A similar kind of faint can occur in injuries or overexertion resulting from increased vagal nerve tone. (The vagus nerve helps regulate heart rate.) People so affected get faint and look "shocky," but they have a *slow* pulse. Usually lying down and resting is the only treatment necessary. If you've ever gotten faint while having blood drawn you'll recognize the syndrome.

One of the most common disturbances runners experience is *shin splints.* The term, which probably derives from the world of trainers and professional athletes, is inexact and may cover a number of related injuries. Where shin splints shade off into actual *stress fractures* of the leg is not certain. The typical shin splint is a pain in the front portion of the lower leg. It is much more common in those runners who run long distances on hard surfaces, like pavement. There is often a specific point of tenderness in the shin, either in the muscles or bone. The pain, which typically occurs when running, is usually moderate, not severe, but it is severe enough to prevent running. The problem may be minute muscle tears and associated bleeding into the surrounding tissues. There isn't much space for the blood to occupy, so pressure is exerted on the nearby tissues, causing pain. As we noted, it is hard to say where a shin splint ends and a stress fracture begins. Stress fractures are small cracks in the tibia (the larger of the two bones of the lower leg), which are usually—again—painful enough to prevent running. Two reasons they are not more readily diagnosed are (1) many people with shin complaints don't bother to get X-rays and (2) often a fresh stress fracture won't show up on the X-ray but will be easier to see when it is in the healing stage, as new bone is being deposited. (Some specialists now perform radioactive isotope bone scanning to detect early stress fractures.) The treatment for both shin splints and stress fractures—two kinds of the overuse syndrome—is rest of the leg, sometimes (in the case of the fracture) for several weeks, possibly the use of crutches.

Hip injuries are not uncommon and are sometimes associated with overuse and sometimes caused by unequal leg lengths with a resulting tilt of the pelvis. This problem, which can usually be corrected with a lift placed in the shoe, should be diagnosed and treated by a sports medicine specialist.

Back problems—muscle spasm, irritation of the sciatic nerve (which arises in the spine and supplies the leg), or a true disc syndrome (protrusion of the disc material between the vertebrae of the back, causing nerve irritation)—can be aggravated by running. The treatment is bed rest on a firm mattress, possibly for several weeks. Since running is associated with a tendency to jarring impact as the foot falls on the running surface, running can increase already present pain and spasm in the lower back. Also, it doesn't really strengthen your back as, for example, swimming does. Runners with poorly developed back structures should consider adding swimming or calisthenics designed to assist the development of the muscles associated with the spine, the abdomen, and the buttocks.

A fairly common occurrence in long-distance runners, and in some other sports as well, is blood in the urine (hematuria). While this is usually microscopic in amount, and not noticed by the runner, sometimes large amounts of visible blood can be passed. Ordinarily this would be reason for an intensive medical workup, but sports medicine specialists have now had enough experience with this finding to recommend that a person with hematuria avoid exercise for forty-eight hours. If the bleeding has disappeared, the hematuria can be disregarded. Keeping this in mind will save you a considerable amount of discomfort, expense, and worry. It appears that the bleeding is likely to be due to disruption of the lining of the bladder or some other part of the lower urinary tract, which heals after the appropriate period of rest.

Recently a report of severe skin irritation as a result of allergy to ethyl butyl thiourea, a chemical accelerator in some artificial rubber products used in running shoes, was published. The innersole material that contained this was similar to that formerly used in rubber wetsuits, and has been associated with a similar allergy in divers. Fortunately, the manufacturer has already altered the process and eliminated the chemical. However, this serves as a warning that substances in clothing, particularly if moisture from sweating is present, may cause irritation because of direct chemical action on the skin or allergies to chemicals.

ORIENTEERING

Orienteering is a sport combining running, hiking, and walking. It was born in Scandinavia in the 1890s and became a competition sport in 1900, when the first contest, between two towns in Sweden, was held. Today, there are over 65,000 active orienteers in Sweden, and a recent international match brought together over 10,000 people from more than thirty countries.

Participants use a hand-held compass to find a number of stations, or "controls," on a map of a woods or other area. Orienteering can be performed as a timed event, with graded points for difficult controls. It can be done on cross-country skis, and it has even been performed (over suitable terrain) on bicycles. It is set up as either a team event or a relay sport.

Clothing that can withstand scratching from branches and underbrush and footwear suitable for the area should be worn. You will need waterproof boots if the area is swampy, hiking boots if it is mountainous, or some kind of running shoe for paved roads and paths. A new type of orienteering shoe, resembling a running shoe, but with a cleat sole, is now available.

It is likely that in earlier times people didn't suffer from overuse syndromes as much as we do, simply because walking and running were part of daily life. In some American Indian groups, for instance, in which the nomadic way of life predominated, it was common for most of the tribe to be on foot; if a woman had to deliver a baby, she did so, and then caught up with the tribe by walking. (The horse was unknown to this continent until the Spaniards introduced it, so foot travel was the only means of movement.) Modern, machine-bound societies are rediscovering foot travel, but there are significant costs and some risks involved. Our society cannot engage in a new and somewhat unaccustomed activity without incurring some disabilities, but it seems to us that we should prepare our children and ourselves for a renewed use of our feet and legs. This certainly makes a lot of practical sense in a world in which energy will continue to cost more; it also makes sense as an alternative to the antisocial and destructive effects the automobile introduces into all levels of our lives, from the aggressiveness it engenders in its users to the waste of space and destruction of community life its roadway system requires.

A pedestrian-oriented society would put people above cars. It would allow us to enjoy our surroundings at a pace promoting rather than hindering observation and participation. The most important lesson Bostonians derived from the experience of the Great Blizzard of 1978 was perhaps the realization that a carless society and streets free of foul-smelling exhaust fumes encouraged people to talk with and smile at neighbors and strangers as they *walked* (or skied) to their destinations. Suddenly not only was the car unnecessary, but, as though by design, a new system of public transportation—yellow school buses (whatever *do* they do with them during the day, anyway?)—emerged to take people where they needed to go. The lesson is that the blizzard wasn't the disaster; the car is.

Walking appeals to all people and all ages. Hiking is for those who enjoy the additional challenge of an uphill climb and the surprise of new views. Running may appeal to the loner, perhaps someone who has a streak of compulsiveness. And orienteering draws sports-lovers who want the complexity of running combined with map-reading, calculating, and a competitive outing experience. All of these activities make solid contributions to your level of fitness and develop your natural potential for movement.

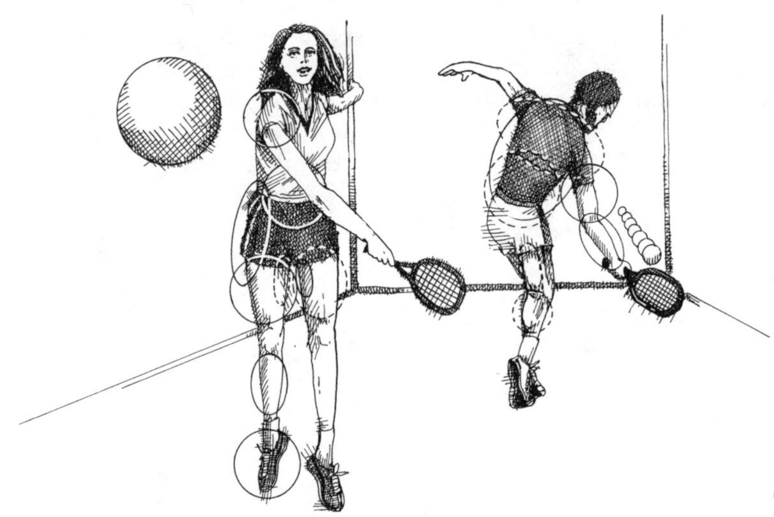

7. Tennis and Other Racquet Sports

Energy consumption:

Doubles tennis	300 cals./hr.
Singles tennis	450 cals./hr.
Racquetball	550 cals./hr.
Squash	630 cals./hr.
Tournament squash	over 660 cals./hr.

Since playing styles vary considerably, there is a lot of difference in calories expended. An inactive game of doubles tennis may utilize very few calories and have little cardiovascular benefit if little running is involved, while a very active game of singles may be an excellent conditioner.

Strengthening effect: shoulder, forearm (or playing arm only), thighs, calf muscles.

Stretching exercises:

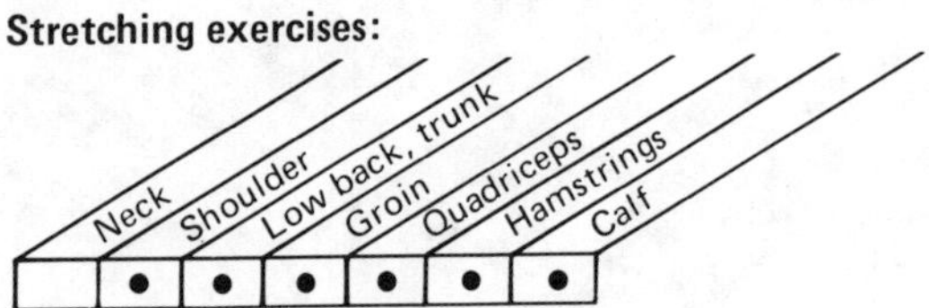

Strengthening exercises:

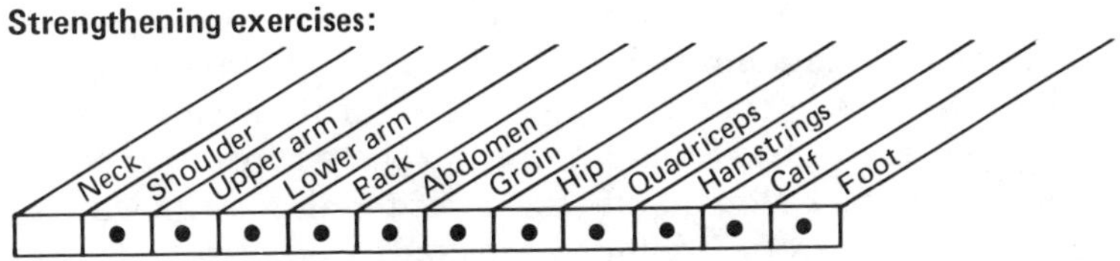

TENNIS, SQUASH, racquetball, and badminton, though quite different in playing environment, technique, and skill demands, place similar physical stresses on their participants and share a common potential for certain types of injuries.

Tennis, the game with the oldest pedigree in this country, has undergone progressive democratization and with it a tremendous growth in popularity. Perhaps because the sport was as often a social outing as an athletic one, there has not been a tradition of specific conditioning or training for it until quite recently. Even now, some respected tennis professionals and instructors deny the need for specific training or even warm-ups before the game and claim that playing tennis is its own best training. However, the existing studies of both professional and amateur tennis players do not support this view. Significant cardiovascular and musculoskeletal stresses can be imposed by the game and imbalances can result.

Racquetball, which is becoming increasingly popular, is claimed to be less technically demanding than tennis. Initially, it is learned more easily, and thus can very rapidly provide the novice with both exercise and enjoyment. Though there has been minimal study as yet of the physiologic demands or injury patterns of racquetball, what has been done shows similarities to other racquet sports.

Analysis of the action aspects of these sports reveals short bursts of muscular activity followed by brief periods of rest—with this alternating pattern extending over a long period of time. Though the primary demands upon the heart and lungs are anaerobic, maintaining a high level of aerobic fitness appears to contribute to the endurance necessary for these games. High levels of aerobic fitness would not be expected from participation in these games alone, and studies of tennis players who do no supplemental aerobic training have confirmed this.

Musculoskeletal demands include repetitive acceleration, deceleration, and impacting of the playing arm by the ball hitting the racquet. Rapid twists, turns, flexions, and extensions of the back and a combination of static (isometric) and dynamic (isotonic) bursts of activity of all the muscles of the lower body, particularly the "antigravity" muscles of the buttocks, front of the thigh and calf, are required. As might be expected, there is a tendency for both these antigravity muscles and their opposing muscles to become tight without a complete stretching program.

Over a period of time the bones, muscles, and ligaments of the regular racquet player actually increase in size and the arm itself elongates. In addition to the extra work done by the arm and shoulder muscles in swinging the racquet, the playing arm must absorb the force from striking the ball. While the potential for a serious injury to the arm from the impact of racquet and ball might seem quite small, recent studies have demonstrated that these accumulated forces are capable of breaking bones or tearing muscles and tendons if proper training and technique are not used.

The playing stance in the racquet sports is a half-crouch, with low back extended and hips and knees held half-flexed. This position places real strain upon the low back and makes it essential to strengthen abdominal, buttock, and thigh muscles to help take the strain off the low back. The army of weekend racquet players who crowd physicians' offices after throwing out their backs on the courts bears testimony to the stresses placed on that part of the body. Participation in racquet sports at *any* level requires maintenance of both strength and flexibility of the back and torso.

Finally, the variety of muscle tears, pulls, and even

complete tendon ruptures that can result from these games bears testimony to the forces generated. In the rapid changes of direction and twists required, muscle/tendon units are exposed to both external stretch by the change in body position and the internal pull of their own shortening. This combination of forces on inflexible and weak muscles can and often does result in serious injury.

CARDIOVASCULAR TRAINING

As noted above, the primary demands on the cardiovascular system by the racquet sports are of short duration, and sprint- or burst-type running is the best training. This short-distance running can be combined with agility drills, such as running from one side of the court to the other and bending forward to touch the side line each time.

Increased aerobic fitness appears to improve endurance for these sports. Aerobic and anaerobic training can be combined in sessions of interval training several times a week. Playing tennis against a backboard, or unopposed racquetball or squash is useful for improving game skills and agility and contributes to anaerobic fitness. A twenty- to thirty-minute jog at moderate speed followed by twenty to thirty minutes of unopposed play, done twice a week, can do much to maintain or improve basic court fitness.

MUSCULOSKELETAL TRAINING

Both strength and flexibility of the upper extremities, especially of the playing arm, are essential. There are two different types of arm strength required. Isometric muscle strength is necessary to avoid injury from the recurrent impact of ball against racquet, while dynamic muscle strength is required for both ground strokes and serves. In particular, a systematic strengthening program for the shoulder and forearm muscles will improve play and help prevent such common afflictions as tennis elbow or shoulder tendinitis. Either free weights or machines can progressively strengthen these muscles in a dynamic fashion, while isometrics can be performed either with the opposite arm in a static resistance, or with the use of certain devices specifically designed for the racquet sports, including the Nautilus forearm strengthener or the Bullworker.

Strengthening the muscles of the low back, flanks, and abdomen using bent knee sit-ups, leg lifts done alternatively with the legs together and spread apart, and bridging exercises should be sufficient exercise. These can be supplemented with either Nautilus or Universal Gym dynamic exercises.

Strengthening the muscles of the lower leg is done primarily with dynamic techniques. In addition, the quadriceps muscles on the front of the thigh and the "dorsiflexion" muscles on the front of the lower leg have isometric demands placed upon them in the stance position and should be strengthened both dynamically and isometrically. A simple isometric program for strength in the thigh muscles is the "wall sitting" exercise described for downhill skiing, while isometric strengthening of the ankle dorsiflexors can be obtained and maintained by simply walking on the heels for progressively longer periods of time each day. For dynamic strengthening of the leg muscles, we feel the use of a Progressive Resistance Program with free weights or one of the exercise machines is best.

While a general program of stretching exercises is necessary for the twisting and turning actions of the racquet sports, flexibility of the low back and abdominal and pelvic muscles is particularly important. Certainly flexibility of these muscles not only helps guard against back strain but also significantly improves playing skills. Flexibility of the calf muscles is also of major importance. The slow stretch techniques described in chapter three are recommended as a part of every training session and warm-up.

INJURIES

Eye injuries from racquet sports are a cause of real concern, both in those games where the opponents are separated by a net (tennis and badminton), and those in which the opponents share the same playing space (squash and racquetball). With net sports, the primary source of injury is the ball or shuttlecock. In countries where badminton is a major competitive sport, shuttlecock injuries to the eye are common, and the hazard must not be minimized. When played well, it is a fast and slashing game. In squash and racquetball, the racquet and the body of the opponent are additional threats. Because of these added risks, eye protectors are recommended. They are available with industrial plastic lenses in frames that can withstand ball impact or racquet blows.

Shoulder injuries from the racquet sports are usually the result of acute or chronic strain of the small muscles along the inner edge of the shoulder joint. These are called the *rotator cuff muscles.* These muscles help hold the joint together and are responsible for the fine adjustments of motion in throwing or racquet swinging. They can be irritated by the constant motion of a weak shoulder. While injuries to these muscles can occur in any of the racquet sports, particular care must be taken by the racquetball player or squash player. The great variety of shots done at all angles, using the sidewalls and ceiling, can result in trapping of these muscles. The best way to prevent rotator cuff shoulder injuries is to maintain proper flexibility about the shoulder through regular stretching techniques, proper warm-up, and dynamic shoulder strengthening exercises that put the shoulder through a slow strengthening motion in front, to the sides, and backwards. In particular, it appears to be advantageous to perform these strengthening exercises while the arms are held close in to the body.

Injury to the elbow is the bane of the racquet sports, particularly tennis. The majority of these injuries are injuries to muscle/tendon units that extend from the fingers and wrist across the forearm to the inner or outer sides of the elbow. Overstretch or overwork of these muscles often can be experienced as sudden sharp pain at the inner or outer edge of the elbow. Sometimes, however, these muscle strains come on slowly and insidiously and will be noted the day following a vigorous game. The increased prevalence of this injury in tennis compared to other racquet sports comes from the extra force on the arm from the larger racquet, heavier ball, and more forceful swing.

Once a player has developed tennis elbow, particularly its more common variant on the outer side of the elbow, it can be one of the most difficult sports injuries to treat successfully. Antiinflammatory medications, cortisone injections, forearm bands, and various combinations of different racquets and stringing techniques are used, but the pain will often recur with serious play. Interestingly, we have often found prominent weakness of not only the forearm muscles in these injured athletes, as expected, but also of the shoulder muscles. The combination of a brief period of overuse without proper warm-up, inadequate playing technique (including "wristiness" on the backhand), and relative weakness of the shoulder muscles appear to set the stage for tennis elbow.

But prevention is possible. It includes regular strengthening and flexibility exercises for the shoulder and forearm, proper hitting technique, and use of a racquet matched to one's level of skill—in recreational tennis, this may be a racquet with large grip, flexibility, whether of wood or metal, and a large "sweet spot." Such a racquet decreases the percentage of balls that hit the outer margins of the racquet and induce potentially injurious sudden twists.

Injuries to the calf muscles and heel cords are extremely common in the racquet sports. They are so prevalent, in fact, that one of them has been dubbed "tennis leg." It consists of a tear of the inner side of the calf muscle—usually from turning to strike a sudden backhand.

The heavy demands placed upon the calves by all the racquet sports put these muscles at special risk. Of all the complete tears of the heel cord that we have seen, more than half have occurred in squash, tennis, and racquetball. Since those injured are mainly weekend athletes over the age of thirty, it has been suggested that the tears may be the result of a simple weakening of the tendon structure from aging. We tend to doubt this. Informal questioning and examination suggest that players who do not regularly train, warm up, and, in particular, those who appear to have tight heel cords prior to injury, are much more likely to injure their heel cords. Once again, there is no substitute for a regular slow-stretch flexibility program.

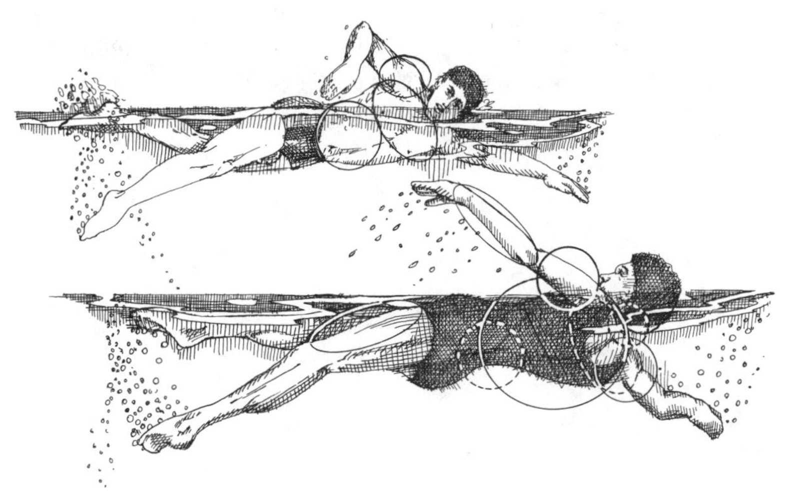

8. Swimming

Energy consumption:

Breast stroke:	450 cals./hr.
Back stroke:	450 cals./hr.
Crawl:	800 cals./hr.

Strengthening effect: shoulders, upper arms, chest, back, abdomen, thighs.

Stretching exercises:

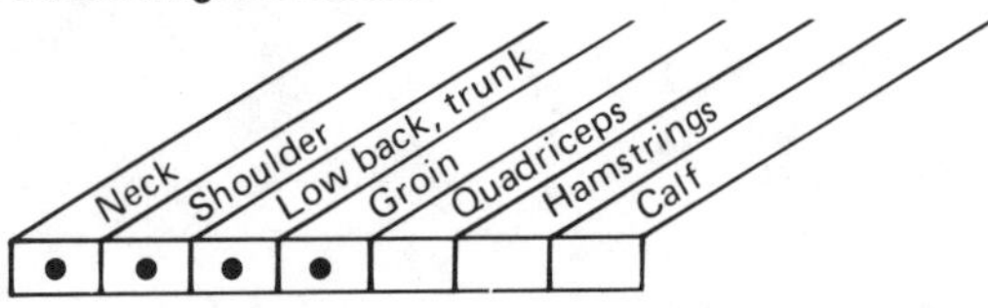

Strengthening exercises:

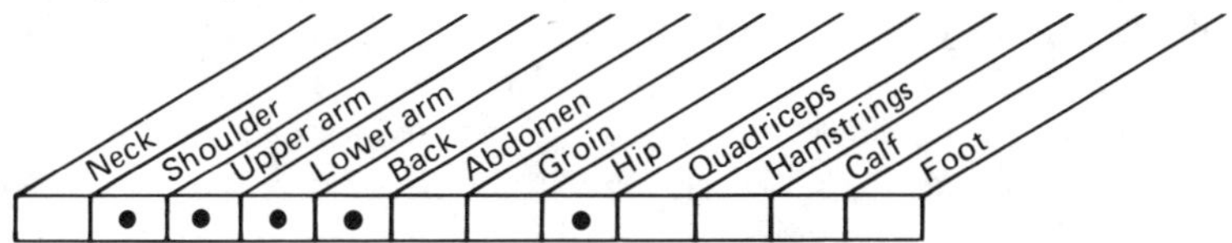

Additional warm-ups: jumping jacks, torso and lower leg stretch, shoulder roll, slow swim.

FOR PRESENT-DAY HUMANS—*homo sedentarius*, as Per-Olof Åstrand has called the species—swimming is a close to perfect antidote to the ailments and stresses caused by urban life. Relatively free of the effects of gravity, a superb solitary venture, and a stimulus to many essential muscle groups, swimming offers its users a way of getting superior muscular and cardiovascular results from a relatively small investment of time. When measured against the results, particularly those affecting the health of the community at large, it is difficult to find any argument against building swimming pools that are available to everyone in neighborhoods, schools, large factories, and office buildings. A national effort along these lines would probably have a significant impact on the current high rate of lost workdays from back trouble, since swimming, of all the sports described, has more positive effect upon the back than any other. In addition, swimming is at least as efficient as running from a cardiovascular point of view and subjects its users to fewer strains and other injuries. It would be ideal as a national life sport.

After an eclipse that began during the Middle Ages swimming re-emerged in the nineteenth century in Europe, consisting of only two strokes—the breast stroke (which is still widely taught as a basic technique in Europe) and a peculiar form of upright swimming something like treading water. The major breakthrough was the trudgen stroke, introduced in 1893 by its namesake (usually misspelled trudgeon) and based upon a double-overhand stroke used in South America. With arms alternately lifted out of the water, drag is reduced, resulting in the fastest-known method of recreational swimming. Because of the stroke's efficiency, fatigue is less of a factor than in some other strokes. Further refinement of the trudgen into the familiar crawl occurred in 1900, when Richard Cavill of Australia introduced a stroke he had observed in the Solomon Islands. The word "crawl" first appeared in an early newspaper article describing Cavill as "crawling" over the water. Cavill's original technique called for only two kicks per stroke, but a variety of refinements, suggested principally by American coaches, developed four-, six-, and even eight-beat kicks. Thus, the leg action shifted from being purely a method of keeping the lower half of the body suspended into one assisting in the drive forward.

Very high oxygen uptake scores have been recorded in swimmers. The aerobic principle of involving many muscle groups in a sport is particularly well served by swimming—the scores of competitors rank as high, for example, as those obtained by competitive runners and cross-country skiers. One factor, however, that sets swimming apart from all other sports is the effect of water pressure on the breathing mechanism. This leads to a slightly less free expansion of the lungs during exertion. Thus long-distance swimmers may have to rely on anaerobic mechanisms for assistance as well as the usual aerobic processes. Certainly more anaerobic training is called for in swimming than in such sports as cycling, running, and skiing.

When men and women swimmers have been compared, women have had more mechanical efficiency at any given speed. Their greater buoyancy, which results from the higher percentage of fat, undoubtedly contributes to this.

From the cardiovascular aspect, recreational swimming with a heart rate of, say, 140 to 150 beats per minute, will burn from fifteen to seventeen calories per minute. A thirty-minute workout, then, will burn almost 500 calories, while strengthening the heart, lungs, and important back support muscles.

In addition to improving the back-support muscles, swimming strengthens the chest and shoulders. As these areas are undergoing development, you may feel some discomfort in your chest. This can be confused with chest pain from other causes. One way of determining whether there is anything to worry about is to press hard on the area in question, or grasp the pectoral muscle where it attaches to the shoulder, just above the armpit in front. If there is tenderness there, it's most likely an effect of stretching and, perhaps, overuse—not a heart attack. If there is still a concern about the source of the pain, consult a physician.

MUSCULOSKELETAL TRAINING

While weight training has proven useful to competitive swimmers in improving performance, the recreational swimmer will not require specific weight training unless he/she develops certain problems. Most problems—and there are remarkably few in this sport—center on the shoulder area.

Painful shoulders, from whatever cause, can be at least partially prevented by a few simple stretching maneuvers.

1. Hanging from a bar by your hands is an excellent way of stretching the shoulder muscles. Do it for as long as you feel comfortable, then repeat a half dozen times.
2. Arm and shoulder flexibility exercises, carried out before entering the water, can be helpful. Stretching backward, because of the need for this motion in the recovery portion of crawl and butterfly strokes, is recommended. Backward stretching, free-swinging forward and backward "windmilling," horizontal swinging, and overhead stretching are all good for loosening up the shoulder.

You can do more comprehensive stretching and strengthening exercises if you feel you are going to aim for greater speed and become involved in competition. However, if your aim is to condition yourself, enjoy the feel of your body in water, and appreciate the sense of relaxation, accomplishment, and tranquillity that a thirty-minute swim will provide, then these simple loosening-up exercises, followed by a refreshing swim, will fulfill your needs. If you haven't been used to doing the crawl, your best bet is to start with a breast stroke (perhaps you will want to get some help from a swimming instructor) and prepare to enjoy one of the world's oldest and most satisfying forms of physical activity.

INJURIES

Although swimming is remarkably free of external hazards as well as sports-related injuries, most of the medical problems associated with this activity are confined to the skin. *Swimmer's itch* is an allergic reaction to the presence in fresh water of a parasite, one of the schistosomes that uses muskrats and certain migratory birds as intermediate hosts. Repeated exposure to the parasite, which in humans superficially penetrates the skin, eventually results in an itching rash that lasts about three days. Treatment calls for calamine lotion and antihistamines. *Swimmer's ear* is an irritation of the ear canal that often begins as a fungus infection and sometimes turns into a bacterial one. Fungi are found everywhere in the environment but cause problems only when certain conditions are appropriate: moisture, enough warmth to allow them to grow, and (often) a dark place. Parts of the body that admirably serve this purpose are the spaces between the toes, the crotch, and the ear canals. After swimming it is a good idea to dry the ear canal. Remember that insertion of any object into the ear is potentially hazardous to the vital eardrum at the end of the canal. The best technique for drying is the application of a small amount of rubbing alcohol that will evaporate quickly. *Swimming pool bacillus* is an organism related to the tuberculosis bacillus (but without the serious potential that organism harbors) and can reside in pools and some other bodies of water. If the skin is broken—perhaps against a rough concrete projection on the side of the pool—the bacillus may enter, causing a chronic sore that can take up to two years to heal. The problem usually requires no treatment, as the sore is often small and insignificant. However, if the bacillus is found in a pool, the water should be drained and the pool disinfected. *Swimmer's shoulder* is an overuse syndrome not confined to swimmers but found in any activity demanding an overhand swing, such as the crawl or certain tennis and racquetball motions. (The rotator cuff of the shoulder can catch on the undersurface of one of the ligaments, causing pain.) As in most of these syndromes, rest, heat, and perhaps an antiinflammatory drug will usually bring about a cure.

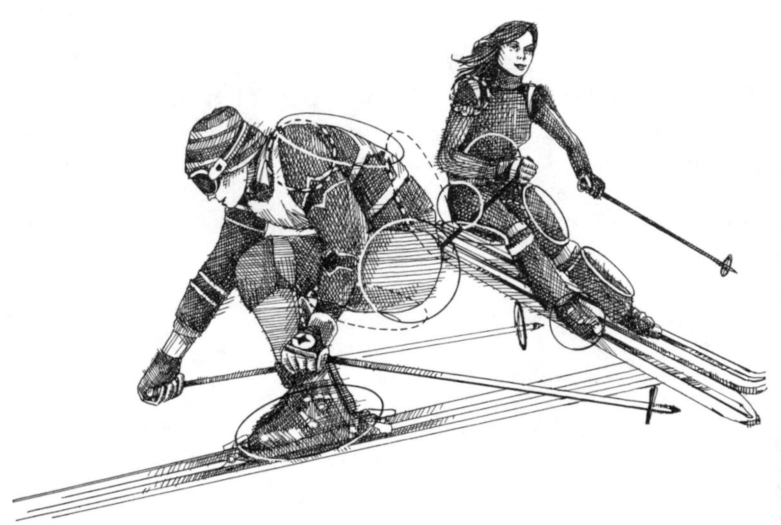

9. Downhill and Cross-Country Skiing

DOWNHILL SKIING

Energy consumption: vigorous downhill skiing consumes 500 to 600 cals./hr.

Strengthening effect: legs, arms.

Stretching exercises:

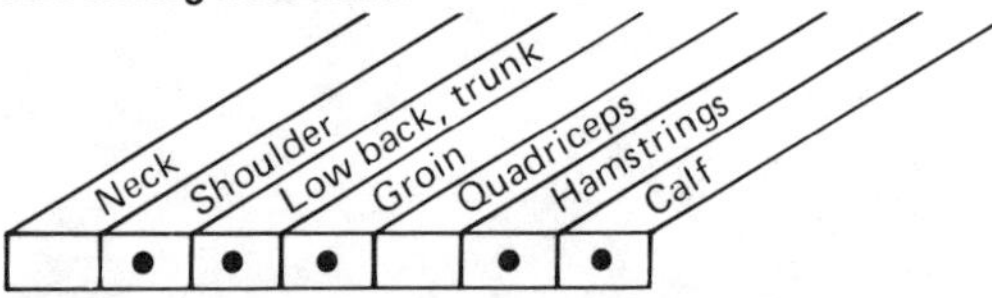

Strengthening exercises:

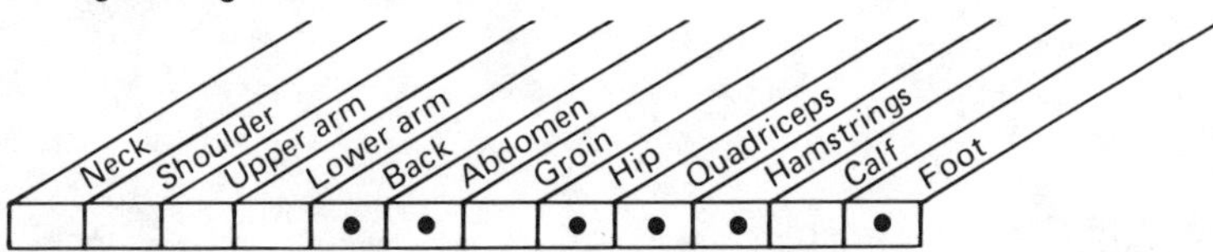

Energy consumption: ranges from 10 to 20 cals./min., or 600 to 1200 cals./hr., thus placing it in the top rank of energy-consuming exercises. However, precise figures cannot be given, as they can in running or cycling, since environmental conditions, the variations in terrain, and factors related to the training and skill of the participants affect the results.

CROSS-COUNTRY SKIING

Strengthening effect: shoulders, back, arms, abdominal muscles, legs.

Stretching exercises:

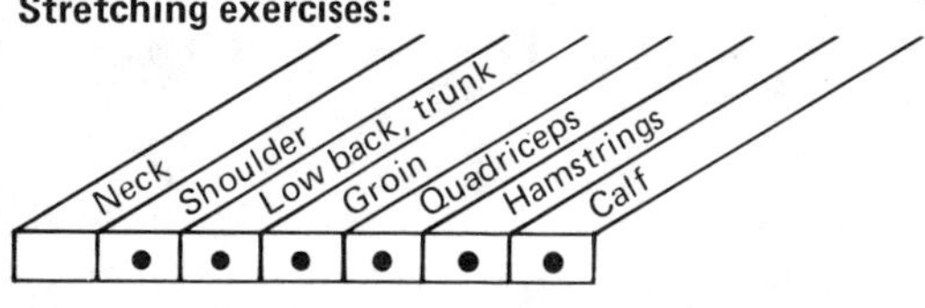

Strengthening exercises:

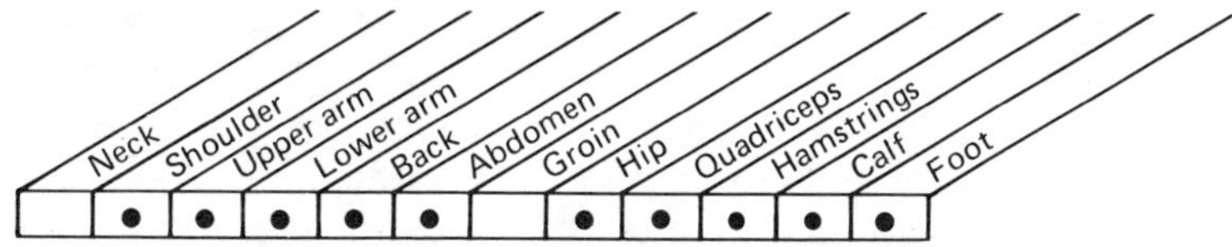

Additional warm-ups: sliding back and forth on skis, rotating trunk at the hips several times.

IN THIS COUNTRY, both downhill and cross-country skiing are now enthusiastically pursued—and while downhill, or Alpine skiing, has the older pedigree here, cross-country skiing is far older worldwide. The beginnings of American downhill skiing are recorded in the hills of southern Vermont at the turn of the century. Early enthusiasts tramped up the slopes and then navigated back down on eight-foot skis clamped to hiking boots. Even the most fit of these early Alpine skiers could manage no more than three or four runs in the course of a day. The dramatic growth of Alpine skiing has been sparked by sophisticated skiing equipment, fast uphill lifts, and skiing areas easily accessible to population centers.

We have seen cross-country, or Nordic, skiing almost catch up with the popularity of Alpine skiing in the past five years. Part of the increase is attributed to Alpine skiers who have been put off by growing lift lines and spiraling ticket prices at Alpine areas. Other converts have emerged from the ranks of such endurance sports as running or cycling, their aim being to continue endurance training through the winter months.

Whatever the motivation, both Alpine and Nordic skiing are now enjoyed by millions of North Americans. While both forms of skiing use skis and poles, the physiologic demands, training preparation, and risk of injury differ significantly.

DOWNHILL SKIING

Nothing can be more enjoyable than a fast, skimming first run down the mountain in new snow nor can anything be more devastating than an awkward, twisting fall in the late-afternoon shadows as fatigued muscles and an exhausted neurological network fail to respond to the need for precise turns and stops. Physical fitness enhances skiing technique, and good skiing technique, in turn, helps prevent injury in downhill skiing. (As Dr. Arthur Ellison, who filmed more than 2000 skiing falls, observed, "He who does not fall down rarely gets hurt.") In the past, though preseason and in-season physical conditioning have been advocated for effective and safe skiing, there has been little agreement on specifics. Activities as diverse as boxing, bicycling, mountain climbing, and roller skiing have been recommended to build fitness for skiing.

As in so many sports, only very recently have studies been done to assess the specific requirements of Alpine skiing. Studies of competitive skiers in peak form indicate that downhill skiing is a combination sport: it requires high levels of both aerobic and anaerobic fitness for high performance and fatigue resistance. The Alpine skier must be both a distance runner and a sprinter. Similarly, the muscle fitness of the lower extremities must combine both isometric and dynamic strength and endurance. In one study, skiers demonstrated the highest isometric thigh muscle strength of all athletes tested. In addition, dynamic "jumping strength" in skiers was surprisingly similar to that of volleyball and basketball players.

These findings seem consistent with the physical demands of downhill skiing. Although sustained, isometric contractures of thigh, calf, buttock, and back muscles are used to maintain body position and control in the descent, intermittent brief bursts of power and dynamic muscle contractions are required to carve turns and the "down-up-down" rhythm over moguls. (Moguls are hillocks of snow that result from the carving action of skis on steep hills.) The need for these two different types of muscle strength and endurance for skiing can be dramatically experienced in spring conditions, where, after several hours of skiing, the skier may still be able to ski effectively and comfortably on a groomed slope but may be totally unable to handle moguls covered with "corn snow" because his/her capacity for dynamic strength, with rapid thrusts and coiling of the legs, has been exhausted by the heavy spring snow.

Cardiovascular Training

The combined aerobic and anaerobic demands of Alpine skiing can be addressed in a variety of ways. Jogging, swimming, or cycling, part of a general aerobic fitness program, should be supplemented with intermittent anaerobic training. Interval training with alternate intervals of jogging and running is an excellent and safe technique. A variant of interval training called *fartlek* training (literally "running play") has been used in Scandinavia for training in such sports as skiing. In *fartlek* training, the athlete varies the basic distance running program with intermittent sprints to an object along his/her path, such as a bush or a rock, and then resumes his/her running pace. With this technique, both aerobic and anaerobic training are accomplished, while motivation and interest are maintained.

Two other techniques have been used to attain cardiovascular fitness for skiing. Jumping rope places important cardiovascular stress on the body over a short period of time. Because it is a strenuous exercise, slow, gradual increases in the length of training are recommended. You should initially jump for only two minutes at one time, with increases of two to four minutes per week per season as fitness and stamina grow. Jumping rope, conveniently done just about anywhere, including home or office, improves balance and agility, both assets in skiing. The strength and endurance of the calf and thigh muscles are also improved by jumping rope, particularly if you use the two-legged jump.

The other exercise that can provide short-burst cardiovascular training, agility, and strength training, is the bench jump, or side jumpover. To do this exercise, stand beside an object such as a cardboard box (about four inches high and eight inches wide) or a large sponge and jump back and forth over it until you get tired. Ski poles can be used to assist in balance, weight transfer, and upper body coordination. As fitness improves, you can use progressively larger objects and increase the duration of the activity.

Musculoskeletal Training

As noted above, the primary demands of skiing appear to be both isometric and dynamic strength of the thighs and lower torso. Static and dynamic strength of the lower legs, chest, and shoulders are next in importance.

The time-honored technique for developing isometric strength of the thighs and the pelvis is the wall-sitting exercise, in which you balance yourself against the wall with your hips and knees flexed at right angles. As you begin this exercise you will be impressed by two things: the surprisingly short period you can maintain the position and the rapidity with which you can increase your endurance—usually five to ten seconds per day.

Another useful exercise for the thigh is isometric setting of the quadriceps with the knee held at a number of different positions from 90 degrees bent to full extension. Your opposite leg is used to provide resistance, and the muscle set is held for seven to ten seconds.

You should do bent knee sit-ups several times a week to strengthen the lower abdominal and hip muscles, which are so important in maintaining body control and balance.

In addition to training to meet the specific muscle demands of skiing, it is also important to strengthen the bones, muscles, and ligaments to increase resistance to impact or twisting injury. One's legs can be exposed to short periods of twisting force before a ski binding releases—or fails to release. Despite the introduction of plastic ski boots, which now provide better protection for the ankle and lower leg, high twisting forces can still break bones or tear ligaments in the leg, unless bones, ligaments, and tendons are made stronger by a specific strengthening exercise. We therefore recommend a good dynamic weight program using either Nautilus, Universal, or free-weight techniques to help maintain the strength of ligaments and muscle/tendon units about the knees, shoulders, and wrists. Recent studies of ski injuries have shown that sprains of the ligaments of the knee—not lower leg fractures—are now the most common serious leg injuries from skiing, while injuries of the upper body, particularly to the shoulders, elbows, and thumbs are occurring much more frequently. Thus, the need to strengthen these areas is clear.

As with muscle strength and endurance, flexibility of the muscles and joints of the lower back, thighs, and lower legs must be maintained by regular stretching exercises. Again, slow stretching is recommended, your peak stretch being maintained for eight to ten seconds.

The quadriceps, or muscle in the front of the thigh, the hamstring muscles at the back of the thigh, and the hip muscles and ligaments require regular stretching. In addition, stretching of the back, lateral torso, groin, and calf muscles can help prevent injury, while improving performance (see chapter three and the Appendix).

Additionally, you can do a brief period of stretching as a warm-up before each ski run. While standing on your skis with the top buckles of the boots unsnapped and the ski poles planted in front for balance, slowly slide your skis backward away from the poles, keeping your knees, buttocks, and back straight. You can also do lateral trunk stretches and trunk rotations while standing upright on the skis.

Injuries

The chance of sustaining injury in downhill skiing, though considerably greater than in cross-country skiing, is no higher than in many other recreational sports activities. If the recreational skier follows a few basic guidelines to decrease the risks, he/she can participate with little fear. A recent study of Scandinavian skiers found that while in a single season 0.02 percent of cross-country skiers injured themselves, only 0.6 percent of downhill skiers were hurt. While it is clear from these figures that cross-country skiing is much safer than downhill skiing, it is also evident that downhill skiing compares very favorably with gridiron football, where the injury rate is 40 to 50 percent of participants per season.

A number of studies of skiing injuries have now been carried out in this country and Europe, and though there may be some disagreement over the relative importance of certain risks, most of these studies show that there are three major sets of factors: (1) skier factors, including age, experience, level of skill, fatigue, and physical fitness, (2) equipment factors, including length of skis, type of poles and boots, the presence of an antifriction device, and the condition of the release binding, (3) skiing conditions, including type of slope, degree of congestion, condition of snow, and time of day. Of these various factors, the most important appeared to be the experience and fitness of the skier and the setting and the condition of the ski bindings.

The types of injuries seen in recreational downhill skiing have changed in the past ten years. In the past, fractures about the ankle and lower leg, including the "boot top fracture," were the most common injuries. But more recent reviews of skiing injuries have shown an increase in the number of injuries to the hands and shoulders, and more injuries about the knee. This changing pattern of injuries has been ascribed to (1) changes in boot design—the higher, more rigid plastic boots transfer more force upward to the knee while protecting the ankle, (2) changes in skiing technique—the backward lean and "hotdogging" techniques of today cause a skier to fall backward into the hill, increasing the possibility of injury to his/her twisted arms and shoulders, and (3) the increase in overall average speed of downhill skiing for all levels of proficiency, thus adding to the number of "impact" injuries to both upper and lower extremities. More recent techniques of teaching, particularly the Graduated

Length Method, move the novice skier immediately into parallel turns, which of necessity require a greater velocity. While parallel skiing rapidly increases the skill of the beginner and makes skiing more enjoyable more quickly, it does not increase his/her experience or judgment in handling variations in terrain or skier traffic.

From all this it is evident that a number of rather complex factors are involved in the rate and severity of downhill skiing injuries. But there are several steps you can take to guard against injury.

The first is proper training, both initially and as you go on to slopes of increased difficulty. Be sure you have mastered one series of maneuvers before you try something advanced. Certainly the widespread practice of labeling slopes or runs as to degree of difficulty has been particularly helpful in matching skiers to slope. As you observe these signs, remember that snow conditions vary and can turn an easy run into a challenge even for the experts.

Proper fitness and conditioning for skiing are extremely important in avoiding injuries—both in preventing falls and by making skiers more resistant to injury.

In addition, warm-up at the beginning of each morning or afternoon session, and even at the beginning of each run, particularly if you have had a long lift ride, is important. A short series of forward and lateral stretching exercises plus several side hops or jumps in place can make a big difference.

Proper attention to ski bindings is also extremely important. (It has been found that maintenance is even more important than type of binding in preventing injury.) While bindings that release too easily are as annoying as bindings that do not release with a fall, most studies show that the latter is much more frequently associated with serious injury. A simple test any binding should pass is the ability to release with a sharp blow on the side of the heel from the opposite boot. Additionally, the heel binding should release with a full forced forward bend by the skier at rest. The presence of an antifriction device between the boot and ski surface definitely assists release.

Liberal use of a silicone spray on binding mechanisms, the sole of the ski boots, and the binding surface of the ski is useful insurance.

Finally, in the event of a serious fall, a few simple measures can help reduce the chance of further injury. Cross ski poles or skis above the downed skier. Reassure and keep the injured skier warm. Make no attempt to move him/her until the ski patrol arrives. Under no circumstances should the ski boot or ski clothing be removed. While most skiers are generally helpful in emergencies, it is a good idea to ski with someone you know at all times. Downhill skiing is not a dangerous sport, but assistance in the event of an injury should be available quickly to offset the effects of cold weather.

CROSS-COUNTRY SKIING

In many parts of the country today if there's snow on the ground, there are likely to be cross-country skiers out enjoying it. That's a big change from just a few years ago when Alpine skiing was the only real outlet.

Nordic, or cross-country, skiing derives from an ancient mode of travel across snow. A picture of a skier dating from the eleventh century has been preserved on a rock near Uppsala, Sweden, and some ethnologists say it dates from the Stone Age. The Lapps of the sixteenth century, known to other Scandinavians as Skrid-Finnen, or "sliders," skied on a leather shoe about three feet long, with a curved toe. The Norse god of winter, Ullar, is always pictured on skis.

What has long been a practical way of coping with snow has become a recreational outlet for millions of people fortunate enough to live in a climate with a steady snow cover of at least a few inches. It has also proved to be a superb conditioner. The combination of upper- and lower-body movement provides cross-country skiers with what is probably the most complete form of aerobic conditioning available. (The maximal oxygen uptake of competitive skiers ranks above that of any other athletes measured.)

For the recreational skier, ski touring can be enjoyed

without highly complicated training or planning. An outing provides a pleasant hour or two, or more, on trails through the woods in winter, or on a nearby golf course or field. The sport is almost silent, and the feeling of being out on a cold winter day is exhilarating. Skiers are rarely cold, even in midwinter, since the heat production in cross-country skiing is very high. Indeed, the clothing worn for this sport is much lighter than that worn in Alpine skiing, in which the exertion is often less and a larger part of which is isometric in nature.

Ski touring has been promoted as a safe winter sport, particularly in comparison to Alpine skiing. That's only generally true. It probably *is* safer, but an accurate picture of the actual incidence of injury has yet to be constructed. Ski touring in this country is still in its infancy as a mass sport, and data are not yet collected. It isn't a totally "benign" sport, at any rate, and certain precautions do need to be emphasized.

The demands of cross-country skiing make it absolutely essential that the body's cardiovascular system be in good working order. This is a sport in which the skier could become isolated and be at the mercy of the elements. A broken ski tip, for instance, without a replacement at hand, is like having a broken leg, and a forced hike in waist-deep snow places massive isometric demands on the muscles and can strain the heart. If you are a smoker thinking of ski touring, better give up cigarettes.

Good leg strength is essential, as is upper body development. The arms and shoulders are in constant use in ski touring, and if they have not previously been exercised they may become sore and stiff after a few hours' workout. Uphill climbing with skis requires some arm power above and beyond the simple poling action on flat terrain. A useful exercise for ski touring is to use a set of arm muscle training pulleys or elastic lines attached to a pole or doorjamb. Both swimming and running provide good training for cross-country skiing, and stretching and limbering-up exercises for shoulders, arms, hips, hamstrings, and ankles are excellent preparation for this sport.

Although injuries are not thought to be common, they can occur. As in downhill skiing, they are most likely to happen when one or more of these conditions exist: skiing beyond one's capability, faulty equipment such as poorly fitting bindings or boots, and fatigue. Taking a last run on skis when you are tired, and therefore not as attentive to trail conditions as when you are fresh, can be hazardous. Most important, ski touring requires a relaxed, rhythmic movement. Skiing in a stiff, tense way will make the sport less enjoyable and you'll be more likely to be injured. Your first several hours of skiing—your self-training—should be over easy terrain so that you can learn to relax and enjoy the gliding that is characteristic of the trained skier.

Because skiing is a winter sport, there exists some need for protection against cold, although as noted, far less clothing is required than with downhill skiing. Usually, cross-country skiers avoid heavy down jackets or leggings and get along with a sweater, windbreaker, and a hat and mittens. A knapsack of some sort is usually helpful, since you may wish to remove pieces of clothing and stow them until needed. Remember that in stopping you can become subject to cold injury, either frostbite or hypothermia, particularly if you have been sweating and have gotten your clothes wet. Therefore, clothing should be of the type that allows perspiration to evaporate.

Injuries from ski touring are mainly to the leg and hip. But since the boots are low and soft, as compared with rigid downhill boots, injuries to the leg are much less likely to occur, in general, than they are in downhill skiing. However, injuries resulting from twisting of the leg from falls in deep snow, or on ice, or because of crossing of the tips of the skis, can be major. Occasional damage to the thumb can occur from abnormal forces generated by the ski pole during a fall.

Ski touring will appeal to anyone who wants to be outdoors in the winter. Its great energy requirements will make even the coldest weather seem warm. The combination of snow, quiet, and exertion make this sport an excellent antidote to the midwinter slump. Your investment in equipment is modest, and from then on there's almost no cost for upkeep or fees. Finally, the health benefits are considerable—it's a perfect sport for those whose winters are snowy.

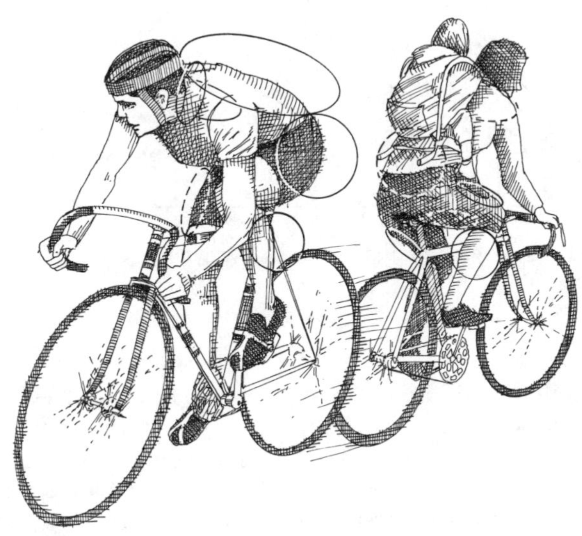

10. Bicycling

Energy consumption:

Cycling	at 6 miles/hr.	270 cals./hr.
	at 8 miles/hr.	330 cals./hr.
	at 10 miles/hr.	400 cals./hr.
	at 11 miles/hr.	450 cals./hr.
	at 12 miles/hr.	550 cals./hr.
	at 13 miles/hr.	650 cals./hr.

Strengthening effect: buttocks, quadriceps, calves.

Stretching exercises:

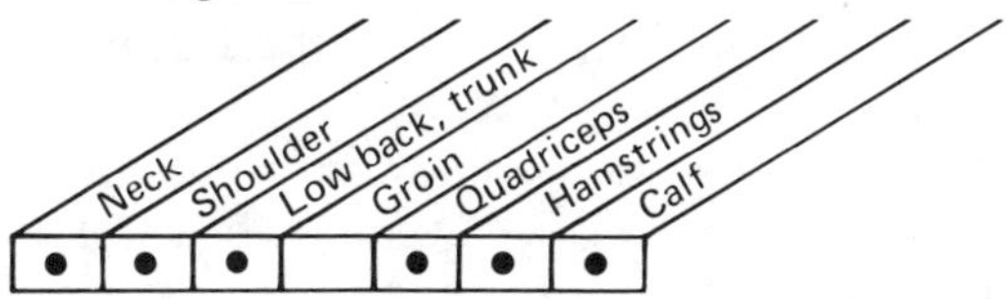

Strengthening exercises:

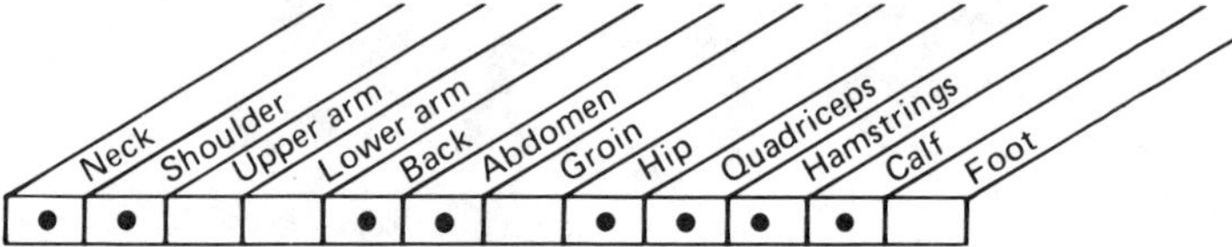

Additional warm-ups: running in place, slow cycling.

BICYCLING REPRESENTS one of the most perfect matches yet devised between the human body and the machine. The mechanical efficiency of the lightweight, multispeed bicycle and its human engine is extraordinarily high compared with other forms of propulsion. The bicycle, which has grown from an early nineteenth-century vehicle using the thrust of the driver's feet against the ground for power, has become a machine of great sophistication and refinement.

The idea of human motion via crank levers and pedals originated in Scotland in 1840 with Kirkpatrick MacMillan of Dumfries. His invention resembled the modern version in basic outline; in addition to the frame, he included a comfortable seat, fancy armrests, and handlebars. This iconoclastic inventor rode his machine for many years and was once arrested and fined for "furious driving" on public roads.

The rotary crank was invented by Pierre Lallement of Paris in 1865. He sold his patent to his employer, Michaux, who set up the first production facility in the world; Lallement then emigrated to the United States and began producing his invention here. Apparently the world was now ready for the bicycle, or velocipede, as it was called, for thousands were sold. All of them belonged to the "boneshaker" class of vehicle, because of the wooden wheels and iron frame construction. At that time there was no way to lessen vibrations and riders became fatigued very quickly. Nonetheless, the boneshaker became extremely popular and set the stage for the development of more advanced types of bicycles.

The American bicycle industry, begun in Boston at the factory of Colonel Albert A. Pope in 1877, quickly became the largest producer of the machines in the world. But when the inevitable slump occurred, British industry reorganized and, finding ways to produce a cheaper model, was for many years the standard of the bicycle industry.

Further developments, using lightweight metals, ball bearings, methods to reduce strain on crucial parts of the frame, and specialized gear ratios have all contributed to the bicycle as we know it today. The highly refined racing bicycle designed in Europe now sells widely in the United States. Today, a large and vocal number of bike riders is devoted to the development of legislation favoring bicyclists' rights, better machines, and the understanding that the bike is a highly efficient, pollution-free, and economical mode of transport.

The bicycle begins to look increasingly attractive as an alternative to gasoline-powered vehicles, at least for short distances and in suitable climates. Its increased use is really an urban planning issue—most cities are poorly adapted to the use of bikes at present. Even if bikeways are not now possible where you live, there is nevertheless room for the development of new and imaginative approaches to foster the use of bicycles. A beginning has been made by the U.S. Department of Transportation, which encourages the development of bike maps and studies relating to cyclists. (Surprisingly, one of their studies on the effect of urban atmospheric pollution on bike riders shows only slight effect.)

Perhaps the way to encourage more bike users starts in the workplace. Most potential users are employed; most people live at some distance from their jobs. Lockers, showers, and a safe place to stow your bike would undoubtedly do more to encourage a bike-commuting society than anything else. If federal tax legislation can provide incentives for the three-martini lunch (thereby fostering restaurant growth), it seems to us that it could do the same for the development of these simple facilities.

Professional biking enthusiasts and their followers who concern themselves with these issues often neglect the powerful argument that really might energize the spread of bike use: health. Cycling not only fulfills most of the criteria for a model community-based commuting system, but it also makes a positive contribution to the health of the population. Since we all pay, through our health insurance premiums and taxes, for the medical care of others, we should have direct concern for the health of everyone in the United States.

Bicycling's positive effect upon the cyclist's health has been well documented and the exercise bike is one of the standard items used for stress testing, along with the treadmill. The bicycle belongs near the top of all the aerobic sports. At a slow pace of six miles per hour on level ground, the rider uses about 300 calories in an hour. Thus, a daily, leisurely three-mile commute each way will burn off the equivalent of over twenty pounds of fat in a year. The extent of the overweight problem alone should be enough to justify a national campaign to get people to use their bikes to go to work.

Cyclists who spend a lot of time on their bikes tend to undergo significant adaptations. Their ability to dissipate heat improves as they become acclimatized, usually after about a week of regular riding. Calorie intake can rise in accordance with energy output (though remember that an excess of calorie intake compared to output will lead to weight gain). Lean muscle mass will increase, while fat will decrease, and the muscles of propulsion, located primarily in the legs, will increase in size and strength.

Bikers tend to develop power in the medial head (on the inside of the knee) of the quadriceps, the large muscle in the front of the thigh. Knee problems, if they do occur, often call for quadriceps exercises designed to strengthen and stretch the muscle and to better stabilize the kneecap. (Runners, in contrast, tend to develop the lateral quadriceps head almost exclusively.)

The biker's muscle development is related to the fact that the knee joint and leg are maintained in a single plane by the requirements of pedaling—compared to the rotational forces affecting runners. Cyclists tend to develop tight hamstrings, requiring good stretching before and after workouts.

Biking problems are often related to the mechanical characteristics of the machine. Pressure on the hand as it grips the handlebar can lead to nerve damage, particularly to the ulnar nerve, which serves the little finger and adjacent portion of the fourth finger. Most injuries of this type can be prevented by wearing biking gloves designed to counteract the pressure. The saddle can be the source of a good many problems. In males, saddle pressure can lead to a numbness of the underside of the penis; in females, the front part of the saddle may rub against the external genitalia, causing severe irritation. Good saddle design is essential, though some problems can be minimized by tilting the saddle enough to avoid rubbing. One solution that has been proposed to avoid the rubbing problem for women is to actually cut a hole in the part of the saddle causing the difficulty, though it would be better if saddles including this modification were already produced. Debate exists over whether there is need to provide a wider saddle for women, because of their wider hip structure. One school of thinking says that this makes no difference to the rubbing problem, though logic would suggest the need for a wider saddle anyway, to provide a resting place for the ischial tuberosities, those "points" on which we all sit. Saddle design is still in its infancy, it seems.

Pain in the muscles of the upper back and neck occur in some cyclists. Often this is related to trying to twist the head around to look backward. The answer is to use a rearview mirror, which can be mounted on a glasses frame or a helmet. In other instances, the pain is thought to be related to the strain of assuming a position over the "dropped" (curved-under) handlebar. To prevent this, adjustments in the height of the handlebar or seat can be made.

Helmets are a necessity for bikers, since statistics show that head injuries account for most of their fatalities and serious injuries. The skull, while a protective box for the brain, is efficient in preventing injury only up to a point—one that can easily be exceeded by the speed of a bike. Lightweight, well-designed helmets are available everywhere, and there is no excuse for not wearing them. They are ventilated, do not obstruct vision, and can save your life.

Since bikes share the roadways with cars, trucks, and motorcycles, it is inevitable that accidents will happen. Most of the time, injuries that do occur are minor and include cuts, abrasions, fractures, and head injuries. Losing control is the principal cause of accidents; this is followed by mechanical or structural problems with the bike. Keep in mind that losing control occurs because of (1) an inability to regain control after hitting holes, bumps, curbs, and similar objects, (2) becoming confused by traffic, and (3) riding the wrong-size bicycle. When structural problems arise they are usually a result of "customizing" of bikes by or for children, or poor maintenance.

Most car-bike accidents have been shown to be caused by the biker; many could have been avoided had traffic rules been observed. At night, the use of reflectorized material on clothing and on the bike, as well as lights, have made an important contribution to accident prevention. Flags have also been shown to be helpful. In this country, the upright flag has been introduced. In Scandinavia, bikers use a short pole attached to the carrier in the rear of the bike that is positioned horizontally so that the flexible staff holds a red triangular flag out toward the traffic passing by. Motorists can see this easily and seem to have an unwillingness to approach it too closely. Since it projects about six inches from the bike, there is adequate clearance for a car to pass without hazard.

A number of states and municipalities have constructed

bikeways to promote tourism. A logical outgrowth of this effort would be the development of the "bed-and-breakfast" tourist accommodations like those now available in England and Ireland. These would be adjacent to the bike paths and would enhance the already existing hostel system. They would encourage more families to travel together and would provide alternatives to the more expensive and less personal motel system.

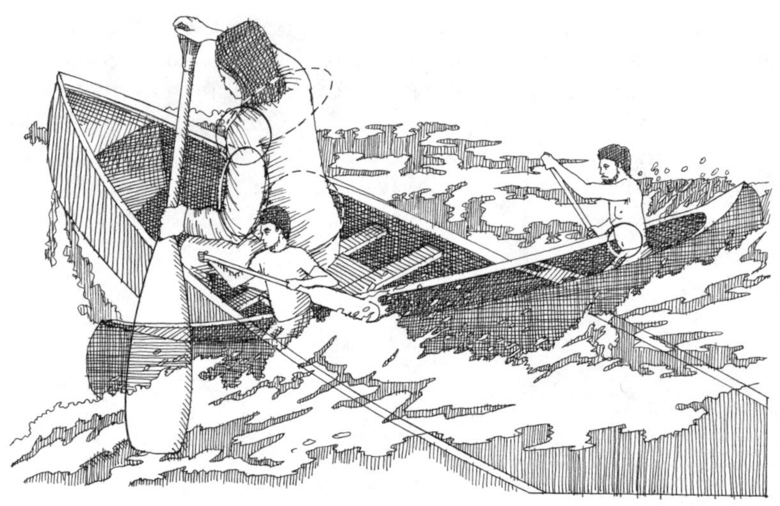

11. Canoeing, Kayaking, Rowing

Energy consumption: quite variable, from about 400 cals./hr. for flat-water canoeing to 800 cals./hr. for vigorous white water canoeing. However the characteristics of white water canoeing and kayaking do not usually permit such sustained effort.

Strengthening effect: arms, shoulders.

Stretching exercises:

Neck	Shoulder	Low back, trunk	Groin	Quadriceps	Hamstrings	Calf
	•	•		•		

Strengthening exercises:

	Neck	Shoulder	Upper arm	Lower arm	Back	Abdomen	Groin	Hip	Quadriceps	Hamstrings	Calf	Foot
Canoeing and Kayaking		•	•		•							
Rowing		•	•		•				•	•	•	•

PADDLING AND ROWING sports have had a long tradition in this country. Columbus, on his first visit to the West Indies, reported encountering natives in large dugout "canoas"—the Arawak name for these craft—capable of carrying a war party of seventy to eighty men. Recent usage defines the canoe as a "boat of long and narrow proportions, sharp at both ends, and propelled by paddles held in the hand, without a fixed fulcrum, the crew facing forward."

The modern kayak, copied from the hide and bone craft used by Eskimo and Northern American Indians, now generally comes in fiberglass and a variety of hull designs, but it still retains the double-bladed paddle with the single occupant facing forward, "wearing" his/her craft.

Versions of both the canoe and kayak have gained wide popularity through the rest of the world, particularly in Europe, where both competitive and recreational craft are common. In Northern Europe, a design called the McFier, attributed to Harry McFie, who returned to his native Sweden from Canada in 1918 and built canvas and cedar canoes, is the most popular recreational canoe.

Both of the paddleboats, canoe and kayak, are used on "flat" water for recreation or "flatwater" racing, as well as on streams with a notable current, so-called whitewater paddling. An International classification of streams or rapids ranging from Class I through Class VI is used to rate the relative hazards of moving water, and sections of many major streams in North America have been given ratings.

Rowing's origins are probably even older than paddling. It employs one of our basic inventions—the lever—to propel the boat through water. The rower usually faces the rear of the boat and pulls a pair of oars, although use of single oars in pairs, such as in college crews, is also common. While an enjoyable outing can be had with any rowboat, the sophisticated singles rowing craft is a source of exercise and informal competition for growing numbers of people. These boats have a sliding seat and fixed footpieces that provide much more efficient use of the entire body in driving the boat through the water.

Cardiovascular Training

Rowing and paddling sports are good examples of the dilemma frequently faced by the recreational athlete. In order to gain maximal fitness benefits *from* the sport, he/she must often engage in certain other fitness activities to prepare *for* it.

Whatever variety of human-propelled water craft you choose, the cardiovascular fitness demands (both aerobic and anaerobic) can be high. While all of these sports, if properly performed, can be used to improve cardiovascular fitness, paddling and rowing are usually not possible on a daily basis and off-water training must generally be used to maintain fitness for satisfactory participation, not vice versa. As a rough guide, the duration of cardiovascular training should be equal to the amount of time you anticipate for rowing or paddling. But this is only a general rule of thumb. Fitness for a whitewater kayak slalom with duration of high-intensity work of three to five minutes is quite different from what is required for a flat-water canoe trip with six to eight hours per day of low-speed paddling.

For either, good aerobic conditioning to provide sufficient oxygen for muscle endurance is essential. This can be obtained from jogging, jumping rope, swimming, or bicycling. If short bursts of sprint-type demands are placed upon the body also, then an interval training program, such as simple jogging of thirty to forty minutes interspersed with short sprints of three to five seconds duration, can be used.

Because participation in many of these sports is, of necessity, of the "special outing" variety, it is imperative to use off-water training sessions to maintain fitness. Even if nothing more than a trip to a nearby boathouse is required for a training session, weather and water conditions, boat repairs and so on will often interfere with a regular rowing or paddling program.

Musculoskeletal Training

Upper body strength and endurance are required in all paddling and rowing. While techniques and body position will, to a certain extent, determine the particular muscle groups to be emphasized, all of these sports are well served by a basic program of upper body strengthening and flexibility.

The foundation of each one of these programs should be dynamic shoulder strength. Bench press, military press (done from a sitting position, if possible), and latissimus dorsi strengthening (done with either the Lat strengthening station of the Universal machine, the Fly and Lat machine of the Nautilus, or with trunk shrugs and dead lifts using free weights) are important.

For kayaking, requiring as it does a great range of shoulder positions, a "complete range" shoulder strengthening program using either hand dumbbells or wall pulleys is recommended. With either device, a series of lifting exercises should be included. With palm facing downward, raise your arm from a position at the side to one of full elevation, repeating twelve to fifteen times. You can perform this exercise at four to six different positions from in front of the chest to the back as the shoulder is rotated about the body.

Strong forearms and wrists are a second requirement for these sports. Exercises that strengthen these parts of the body can be easily performed in a variety of ways. Chin-ups or wrist and arm curls with free weights or machine are all good. Since in certain phases of kayaking and canoeing isometric techniques are used, upper arm isometric setting exercises of eight- to ten-second duration are also important.

While each of these sports puts high demands upon your back, the actual position of the back during the activity and the degree of stress placed upon it vary considerably. In kayaking, your back can be positioned in a stable and low stress posture. With hips and knees flexed and supported, and the use of a support in the midback, there is little chance of excessive force being applied to your back. R. Jay Evans, U.S. Olympic kayaking coach, has seen a number of people with back trouble who have been highly successful in kayaking. He attributes this to the *chaise longue* position of the paddler.

However, in canoeing, significant stress is put across the back and a strong and supple back is important to prevent injury. As you kneel, with buttocks resting against the thwarts, your back is used as a bow, with both back and abdomen contributing to the force of the stroke. Similarly, in rowing, a strong back is essential to coordinate the drive of the legs with the arms and shoulders.

In each of these sports, the dangerous S curve of the back, which means hunching of the upper back and swaying of the lower back, must be avoided, as serious injury may result. A series of simple back exercises that can help overcome this tendency includes sit-ups, leg lifts, pelvic tilts, and slow upward bridging of the back while lying flat upon the floor. These exercises should be done regularly and progressively, in conjunction with back flexibility exercises, both for protection and to increase performance.

In kayaking and canoeing, in particular, flexibility of the upper neck and back in all directions should be maintained. Lateral flexibility, in particular, is required for such maneuvers as bracing, draw strokes, or the Eskimo roll—in which the inverted boat is righted.

Injury Prevention

Warming up before a rowing or paddling session—with particular emphasis on stretching the shoulder and back—is a simple, but too often forgotten, injury preventor. In addition to slow stretching, you should do neck rotations, shoulder and trunk rotations, shoulder thrusts, and a brief series of sit-ups, jumping jacks, or runs in place before stepping into the boat. While these warm-up exercises may not be necessary if transporting the boat to the water has already raised a light sweat, there is no substitute for slow stretches.

Shoulder problems in these sports are of two types: (1) shoulder tendinitis or bursitis, which is usually the result of excessive stress over a short period of time to shoulders that have not been properly trained, and (2) shoulder dislocations, which can occur in whitewater canoeing or kayaking when a sudden twist of the shoulder occurs in a bracing maneuver. The best way to prevent shoulder tendinitis is a muscle strengthening and flexibility program of the entire upper body, along with proper progression of training. As in other overuse injuries, improper training is the single most frequent contributor to injury. Slow, steady increase in duration and intensity of paddling or rowing and a gradual progression in degree of difficulty of the watercourse attempted is the best way to avoid injury.

The prevention of injury in whitewater paddling remains a serious concern. Every year serious injury and death result from the violation of certain basic safety principles. Perhaps the most important of these are proper technique and matching the athlete to the water conditions. This includes, of course, a mastery of basic paddling techniques, including righting a capsized boat, proper physical fitness, and paddling with experienced companions.

Protective equipment should include a well-fitted helmet that covers the temples, is well secured, and has a collapsible liner. You must also wear a proper life jacket, one that does not inhibit paddling but has between fifteen and twenty-five pounds of buoyancy. In addition to assisting in swimming in the event of a tumbling descent in rapid water, such a jacket can provide impact protection to ribs and torso. Specific aspects of safety techniques in navigating a fast stream and in avoiding injury once in the water have been well described in kayaking and canoeing literature and certainly should be consulted.

Paddling and rowing, properly done, can improve your cardiovascular and muscular fitness to a great extent. Muscles of the arms, shoulders, and back are particularly strengthened by these sports. With slow, progressive increase in muscle work, soreness and stiffness can be avoided while strength is increased. Supplemental stretching exercises of the shoulders and back will help insure that you use these strengthened muscles to full advantage. Certainly these sports are one of the best roads to general fitness for the amateur athlete.

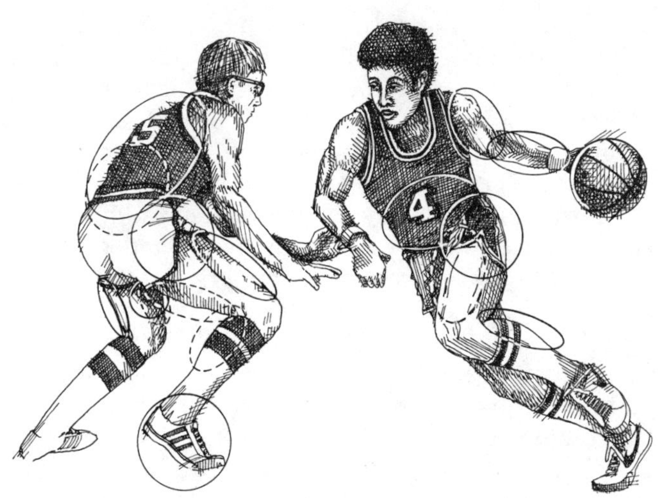

12. Team Sports – Football, Rugby, Soccer, Basketball, Baseball, Softball

Energy consumption: generally, no estimate ot calories can be made for team sports, as there is considerable variability in their style of play and in their demands. Baseball, for instance, may involve little energy output, while basketball, soccer, and rugby, played continuously, may burn 700 to 800 cals./hr.

Strengthening effect: depends entirely upon the sport. Soccer, rugby, and basketball are conditioners for the legs, while basketball has the additional benefit of strengthening arm and shoulder muscles to some extent. Baseball and football, by themselves and without specific training, do not add to muscle strength appreciably; in addition, their intermittency of participation makes them unlikely to be of value.

Stretching exercises:

	Neck	Shoulder	Low back, trunk	Groin	Quadriceps	Hamstrings	Calf
Football	•	•	•	•	•	•	•
Rugby	•	•	•	•	•	•	•
Soccer	•		•	•	•	•	•
Basketball			•	•	•	•	•
Baseball		•	•	•	•	•	•

Team Sports—Football, Rugby, Soccer, Basketball, Baseball, Softball

Strengthening exercises:

	Neck	Shoulder	Upper arm	Lower arm	Back	Abdomen	Groin	Hip	Quadriceps	Hamstrings	Calf	Foot
Football	●	●	●	●	●	●	●	●	●	●	●	
Rugby	●	●	●	●	●	●	●	●	●	●	●	
Soccer	●				●	●	●	●	●	●	●	●
Basketball					●	●	●	●	●	●	●	●
Baseball		●	●	●	●	●	●	●	●	●	●	●

ALTHOUGH INTEREST in sports and recreation in general has had its most visible expression in the unprecedented growth of individual sports and fitness programs for adults, organized team sports are also spreading widely. In the past, team sports for adults were dominated by adult males with a strong tradition of participation in the sport during high school or college. Now recruits frequently are men or women with no previous experience in the sport. Though the skill levels of the returning "old pro" and the enthusiastic novice may be quite different, they share similar needs for fitness training and injury prevention.

Team sports participation provides a special challenge to the adult athlete. This is because the individual player frequently cannot set the limits of his/her own participation according to his/her own fitness or fatigue level, since team pressure to continue play often takes precedence. In addition, the existence of a prearranged season schedule tends to pressure the individual to play when he/she is not necessarily in top shape or is perhaps incompletely recovered from a previous injury. This presents the potential for the serious aggravation of a relatively minor injury, or the occurrence of a new one.

Unfortunately, many amateur athletes are haphazard in their fitness training for team sports. Furthermore, the traditional social atmosphere of many of these sports—with the beer keg at the sidelines—may detract from fitness while significantly increasing the hazards of participation. Poor fitness levels, rusty technique, and a casual approach to sports competition all set the stage for serious injury.

FOOTBALL

Club football can provide an enjoyable outlet for the young adult who wishes to continue in a heavy contact sport after high school or college. But given the contact nature of this game, and the fact that the action lasts for intervals of three to five seconds, the player must specifically train to withstand its impact demands and expect little, if any, aerobic fitness from the sport itself.

Systematic weight training on a year-round basis, even during the playing season (though with lighter weights) is mandatory. The objective should be to strengthen muscles, tendons, ligaments, and bones and increase their resistance to injury.

While an overall program of weight training should be followed, special effort must be made to strengthen the neck, low back, and torso. Frequently, free weight or even machine programs will strengthen most of the muscles of the upper and lower extremities, but not have specific exercises for the neck, back, or torso—which are most in need of protective strengthening for football.

For neck strengthening we recommend an isometric program in flexion, extension, lateral bending, and rotation, with the player, or an opponent, providing resistance. You can do progressive resistance exercises using free weights, the neck harness of the Universal Gym, or the Nautilus neck machines. A trainer for one of the professional football teams told us that, in his estimation, the Nautilus neck machine was the single most important piece of protective equipment owned by his club.

Abdominal and low back strengthening can be done by simple calisthenics—sit-ups and leg lifts—with progressive resistance from weights held behind the head, or from sit-ups done on an inclined bench. Sit-ups are most beneficial if performed slowly and smoothly with the legs flexed up at the hip and knee.

Flexibility is extremely important for football, particularly flexibility of the hamstrings, lateral abdominal muscles, and heel cords; this is due to the rapid acceleration and changes of positions in the game. Systematic stretching programs have been shown to decrease injuries, particularly early-season muscle pulls. The Pittsburgh Steelers have one coach, called "the ballet master," whose sole duty is to insure that flexibility exercises are performed systematically and correctly.

Since the metabolic demands of gridiron football are primarily anaerobic, most attention should be directed to the twenty- to forty-yard wind-sprints. It is the feeling of many experienced coaches, however, that interval training of quarter and half miles should be part of the program.

Since safety in gridiron football is heavily dependent upon protective equipment, properly fitted and maintained equipment is imperative. One of the most worrisome problems of informal football, next to inadequate fitness, is inadequate protective equipment. If the services of a qualified athletic trainer are not available, personnel at sporting goods stores can often provide assistance.

RUGBY

While historically related to football (American and Canadian gridiron football both were derived from rugby), rugby football differs significantly from its descendant. For example, protective equipment, developed to a sophisticated and sometimes dangerous degree in gridiron football, is specifically prohibited in rugby. Unlike gridiron football, with its "plays" and frequent stoppages, rugby is a much more continuous game, akin to soccer, with no time-outs or substitutions allowed during play. Each player is expected to play all of the two forty-minute halves, with a five-minute respite between halves.

A rugby team can be fielded quite inexpensively, and the relative interchangeability of positions gives it a flexibility much like soccer. Although rugby is a contact sport, there is no blocking of opponents, and only the ball carrier may be tackled—and this only to strip him of the ball and continue with play. When properly played, rugby football is a demanding, high-endurance sport with a relatively low rate of injury.

The past five years have seen the addition of women's rugby in many cities and campuses. Initially, injury rates appeared high and concern was expressed as to the relative safety of this game for women. But closer analysis showed that many of these injuries were due to inadequate playing technique and lack of conditioning rather than the contact nature of the game.

Cardiovascular requirements of rugby football are both aerobic and anaerobic. The player must be able to maintain a slow-fast running pace throughout the game, showing good endurance and bursts of sprinting. We have found interval training to be highly successful as a preparation. Two different techniques are used.

In the first, players are asked to run a prescribed course (usually around the rugby field) at a fast jog. Each player should set his/her own pace, a pace at which he/she can carry on a conversation. This jog is interspersed with sprints of ten to twenty yards at maximum speed—obviously without conversation. The jog is then continued following the sprint until the player feels he can resume conversation, at which point he/she sprints again. The duration of this exercise can initially be only fifteen minutes, but as fitness improves it can be kept up for forty minutes. Performed twice a week, this exercise improves the fitness of the entire team, while each player progresses at a rate appropriate for himself/herself.

The second technique that is useful is no contact, "ruck and run," unopposed rugby, where a squad of players moves up and down the field at match speed, simulating passing or running attacks, scrums, or lineouts. Done at a sharp pace, this drill can be valuable in the improvement of cardiovascular fitness, coordination, and game skills.

It should be kept in mind that the potential for neck and shoulder injuries in rugby makes weight training for injury prevention a necessity. In addition, since every player is a potential sprinter and open field runner, flexibility must be maintained, particularly of the hamstrings, groin, and back muscles. Forwards also have to concentrate on strengthening their backs, buttocks, and upper legs. In the off-season, rugby players should strive to maintain a high level of cardiovascular fitness and use a combined endurance and strength program. Alternating days of aerobic and weight training has proven highly successful.

SOCCER

Soccer, or association football, is one of the world's most demanding sports. Its origins are found in nineteenth-century England, where villages played games of kickball against each other with limitless numbers of players, the object being to drive the ball into the opponent's village. This game has evolved into a highly sophisticated and competitive sport that can be played at all ages or levels of skill. Growing rapidly in this country, soccer is a safe and strenuous competitive sport for both men and women. While physiologically an interval sport—like rugby football—it usually requires more continuous running and a higher level of running fitness.

Upper body weight training and strengthening is not as important in soccer as it is in many other sports. It does, however, call for strength and flexibility of the entire spine from neck to lower back. Powerful neck muscles are required for good heading of the ball, while a strong, flexible lower back is essential for the twists and sudden deceleration of dribbling, kicking, and trapping.

It is clear that the most important requirement is a proper balance of strength and flexibility in the legs. The large thigh muscles in the front of the legs provide strength for driving and sudden burst of speed, while the hamstrings at the back of the legs, in addition to powering kicks and leaps, must also have enough flexibility to avoid tears from the extreme stretching demanded in kicking and trapping the ball. While a systematic weight-training program—particularly one directed to dynamic strengthening of the neck and legs—can significantly improve performance, the first priority of the recreational soccer player must be to attain and maintain a high level of flexibility of the major muscle-tendon groups about the hips, knees, and ankles. Second in priority is to maintain the strength and flexibility of the muscles and tendons about the ankle because of the high incidence and often serious disability from ankle sprains and injuries. Third, the strength and flexibility of the low back must be maintained to avoid serious disability.

Cardiovascular training for this demanding game must address both endurance and burst stress. An interval training program, as described in detail for rugby, is ideally suited to soccer. In addition, many of the ball handling and kicking drills of soccer can be used to develop short-burst running fitness while improving game skills.

BASKETBALL

Of all the various team sports available to the recreational athlete, basketball comes closest to fulfilling the basic objectives of any fitness program, and it does so at a relatively low rate of injury. The recreational basketball player can maintain a high level of cardiovascular fitness simply by playing the game, with little need for additional preparation or training. Furthermore, the game can be played easily with almost any number of players and with a great range of skill levels and still provide good exercise for each participant. The interchangeability of positions and informality of participation serve to maximize the exercise benefits for players, since each participant is able to develop the appropriate amounts of overload for himself/herself without risk of overstress.

While an additional weight-training program may enhance performance—particularly jumping ability—it is by no means essential. Once again, the primary emphasis of the recreational basketball player who wishes to avoid injury should be on maintaining lower extremity strength and flexibility — especially about the ankles. Ankle sprains and knee injuries are the curse of the basketball player. The best way of preventing them is to maintain the strength and flexibility of the legs. Opinions vary as to the protective value of high shoes or ankle taping. Ankle taping can be useful in supporting a recently injured ankle that has not yet fully recovered, but there is no substitute for strong, flexible muscles, tendons, and ligaments.

BASEBALL AND SOFTBALL

The team sports that require the most supplemental conditioning are baseball and softball. The potential for serious injury from these games is often unappreciated, probably due to an underestimation of the athletic stress of these games. Lack of fitness in many recreational participants also contributes to a relatively high rate of injury. This is in marked contrast to organized baseball at the school or college level, where the injury rate is low compared to other varsity sports.

Both the cardiovascular and musculoskeletal stress tend to be of short duration. Whether you are turning and running to field a fly ball or moving around the bases after a hit, the cardiovascular stress generally is of only five to fifteen seconds' duration. Anaerobic fitness and training—of the wind-sprint variety—is the best preparation along with a good base of aerobic fitness.

Musculoskeletal demands are of three different types. The recreational athlete is particularly susceptible to overuse injury of the shoulder. This is usually the result of brief periods of excessive arm use without well-spaced training sessions between. Second, the roll call of strained backs, pulled muscles, and twisted necks after the office softball game is often impressive. A sudden twist or reach for a ground ball, an overthrown ball to first base, or a hearty swing can overstretch muscles that have been allowed to become tight and weak or are not properly warmed up before a game. The third source of injury in these games is an occasional ill-advised slide or collision between opponents or teammates during a game. While poor game skills frequently cause these injuries, an additional factor can be the mix of social life and sport that often occurs in these recreational games. The combination of slow reflexes and heightened valor resulting from a few sideline glasses of beer in the hot sun has contributed to many recreational sports injuries.

The recreational athlete, particularly in team sports, must have a proper respect for the athletic activity he/she is undertaking. He/she, just like the college or professional athlete, may be exposing the body to stresses that can result in serious injury if it is not properly prepared and that—far from improving basic fitness—can be harmful because of the intermittent and excessive overload imposed on both the cardiovascular and musculoskeletal systems. Excessive valor and heroics take their toll on unprepared athletes engaging in team sports on an irregular basis.

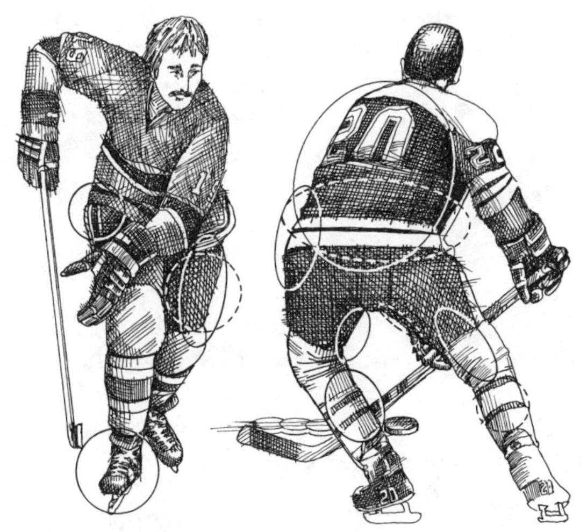

13. Ice Hockey and Skating

Energy consumption: considerable variation exists, from the modest expenditure of recreational skaters to that of champion speed skaters. An average figure of about 500 cals./hr. comes as close as is possible to estimating the value of the sport in these terms.

Strengthening effect: hamstrings, calves, foot, groin.

Stretching exercises:

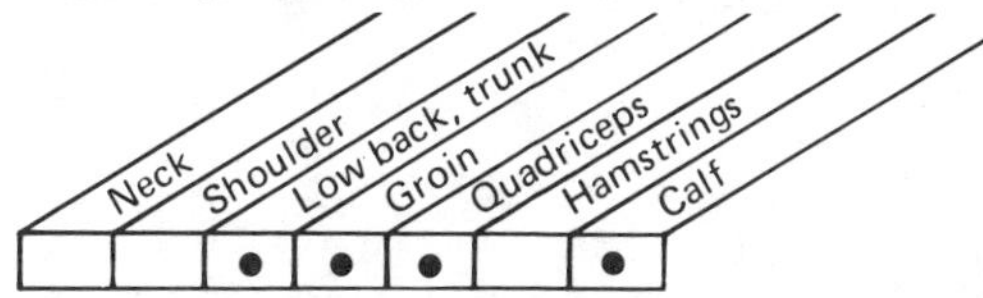

Strengthening exercises:

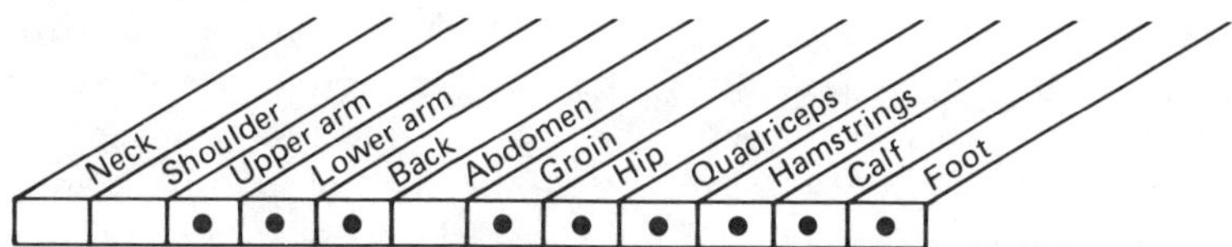

ICE HOCKEY and free skating, which share the same rigid playing surface and use similar footwear, have little else in common. Hockey is a demanding team sport incorporating sophisticated skills and pucks, sticks, and protective equipment. Recreational skating, in contrast, can be performed at whatever level of stress or demand the skater wishes—including systematic endurance training.

ICE HOCKEY

Until quite recently, ice hockey in most parts of the United States was a novelty sport played by Canadian expatriates before unschooled, but enthusiastic spectators. This pattern is undergoing rapid change. Amateur hockey players from six to sixty now vie for ice time at all hours of the day and night throughout the year.

Charles Schultz, the originator of the Peanuts cartoon, plays regularly on a club hockey team in Minnesota that has no member younger than fifty. A friend of ours stopped playing hockey after college and was away from the game more than twenty years; his interest was rekindled watching his two sons and his daughter play the game. Returning to hockey in his early forties, he lost twenty pounds of extra weight in the first year of play and has stayed with the game.

Most adult hockey leagues play with modified rules in which body checking is not allowed. Others allow "brush checking" (screening without impact) but no checking against the sideboards.

Hockey has sometimes been called soccer on skates, and the recreational player, whose limited ice time is devoted to playing in organized games, can pattern off-ice training after soccer. It is a game with high aerobic or endurance cardiovascular requirements, as well as anaerobic, short-burst demands. Interval training, with continuous jogging interspersed with sprints of five to ten seconds' duration as detailed in chapter nine, is highly recommended. The goal is to sustain a brisk jog, with fifteen to twenty interspersed sprints, for a full twenty minutes—the duration of one hockey period. However, players returning to the game after a long interval away from sports should build up with a basic, progressive jogging program for at least three to four months before beginning interval training.

Strong legs have been one of the traditional characteristics of hockey players, but, unfortunately, so have groin pulls. Muscle strength without flexibility can lead to muscle pulls or tears. The recent additions of systematic weight training and systematic stretching are very important to prevent injuries. Power turns, scrambles for the puck, and even shots at goal tend to develop leg muscles with strength and endurance, which, at the same time, can become tight and inflexible unless extra attention is paid to systematic stretching.

Interestingly, recent studies of hockey and skating in general have revealed how important upper body strength is for "power skating." Successful hockey coaches are beginning to stress this in addition to muscle strengthening of the legs and torso. A weight-training system that includes training of the upper body, torso, back, and legs should be used two to three times per week. Particular attention should be paid to building up the strength of your groin, thighs, and ankles. As in all the interval sports where both muscle strength and endurance are required, a complete weightlifting program with seven to ten repetitions of each exercise, repeated three times, is recommended.

In addition to strengthening, overall flexibility will contribute to playing skills and help reduce injuries. Hockey players should concentrate especially on low back, hamstring, groin, and calf muscles. Daily stretching exercises of fifteen to twenty minutes performed at home, in a gym, or at the office can make a significant improvement in flexibility in as short a period as three to four months.

The adult recreational hockey player should take a lesson from younger players regarding the prevention of face and eye injuries. The use of protective helmets and face protectors has now become mandatory for junior hockey players throughout the United States, and a dramatic decrease in the occurrence of serious face and mouth injuries has been seen already. While it may be several years before protective helmets and face masks are required in adult hockey, it is difficult to understand why an adult playing recreational hockey would not use this indispensable protective equipment. No one can afford a serious eye, face, or mouth injury from a misplaced puck or stick. Last year, before helmets and face masks were required in the Junior Hockey Leagues in the United States, more than 25,000 facial injuries were reported. While figures from the past season have not yet been compiled, preliminary reports suggest fewer than 200 injuries.

To many sports physicians, hockey is synonymous with hamstring or groin muscle strains. While most often occurring in a defenseman who extends a leg to block a shot, these muscle pulls can occur in any hockey player and, unfortunately, are seen all too frequently in the recreational player who has not maintained muscular fitness and flexibility.

A game played in a cold environment with rapid twistings and turnings of the body absolutely requires proper warm-up. While a brief period of shots at goal and a few turns around the ice may help get up a bit of a sweat, these are no substitutes for proper stretching exercises. In addition to a skating warm-up, slow stretch of the low back, front and back of the thighs, groin muscles, and calf muscles must be done. A complete set of stretches can be done on the ice with the assistance of nothing more than the sideboards. While grasping the sideboards, you slowly push yourself away from the edge of the boards, maintaining your skates flat on the ice. This provides a slow progressive stretch for the heel cords and calf muscles and should be maintained for eight to ten seconds. Next you rotate your legs outward and position them flat against the sideboards. Maintain this position and slowly go into a half knee bend position. This provides excellent slow stretch to the groin muscles and front of the hips. The third simple technique that can be done on skates is to bend forward from the waist, bend the knees and grab the ankles, and then slowly straighten the knees over a period of eight to ten seconds. Repeating this three or four times provides proper warm-up stretching for the low back and hamstring muscles.

Too many recreational hockey players become negligent in maintaining, or attaining, basic skating technique. A number of the more serious hockey injuries occur with falls that are often the result of poor skating. It is important for the recreational hockey skater to maintain his/her basic forward and backward skating technique with free skating practice sessions throughout the year. While it may seem unnecessary to encourage fundamental skating skills for a sport like hockey, too many recreational hockey players overlook them.

ICE SKATING

Ice skating, in many ways, comes close to being the ideal "carryover" sport, as it can be enjoyed at any level of skill. It is also a sport in which most members of the family can participate.

While skating generally requires little formal cardiovascular preparation, it can itself be used as a source of either endurance or interval training, depending on the structure of the workout. For athletes in training it can be a way of adding variety to a basic fitness program. Certainly alternate days of jogging, swimming, and ice skating provide the ideal fitness program—one that sustains interest and enthusiasm.

While the cardiovascular demands, or benefits, of skating are totally dependent on the duration and intensity of the skating, the musculoskeletal aspects are more specific. Leg strength and endurance, particularly about the ankles, are important. Many otherwise fit athletes have been embarrassed by wobbly ankles and weak thighs after a brief session on skates. If you wish to include skating in your sports program, systematic ankle strengthening, including heel and toe walking, is very important. Another valuable training technique is the use of a balance board—which is nothing more sophisticated than a three-foot section of board balanced on a 4 by 4 post or round log that is free to roll from side to side. Tilting from side to side at increasing rates of speed can build up your balance and strength, including the strength of the important peroneal muscles on the outside of the ankle.

Maintaining flexibility of the legs is as important for skating comfort and safety as is muscle strength. Slow stretching of the calf and heel cords, the hamstring muscles on the back of the thigh, and the groin muscles on the inside of the thigh are as important as the general stretching program (see Appendix).

Skating is an activity much like skiing, in which what injury there is is often associated with falling. Sometimes a person breaks a bone when an outstretched arm or projecting knee strikes the ice. Muscle/tendon injuries are often also the result of a fall or a sudden twist in an attempt to prevent a fall. Two steps can be taken to prevent injuries from falls. The first is to improve skating technique—either by taking lessons or by adjusting speed to one's level of skating. The second is to fall properly, in a relaxed, collected fashion, while attempting to dissipate the impact by rolling with the fall. Clearly proper falling technique in the event of a mishap can make all the difference between an embarrassing fall and a serious injury.

Most of the really serious injuries we have seen from skating have resulted from "unskilled falls," in which a misplaced attempt was made to prevent the fall by reaching for the rink side or a friend rather than by falling in a relaxed fashion and tumbling on impact. By observing a few simple precautions, the recreational skater can safely adapt this sport to almost any level of fitness training.

Ice dancing and figure skating, which are popular at ice skating clubs and commercial rinks, present the added requirements of coordination, synchronized skating, and jumps. The recreational skater who decides to participate at this level must, in addition to refining his/her skating technique, train to toughen muscles, bones, and ligaments to protect them from the greater forces generated by the impact of unforeseen falls. But with proper strengthening and stretching, and progressive skill training, ice dancing and figure skating can be safe and enjoyable additions to any fitness program.

SKATE TOURING

A sport that is growing rapidly in popularity in Scandinavia but that has as yet received little attention in this country is skate touring. Using special, long blades, in some ways analogous to cross-country skis, the skate tourer can travel for miles with relative ease over frozen streams or lakes. Proponents cite fitness benefits equal to cross-country skiing, without the hazards of "downhilling" on cross-country skis. Parts of this country are well adapted to skate touring and it could conceivably enjoy a popularity much like the current boom in cross-country skiing.

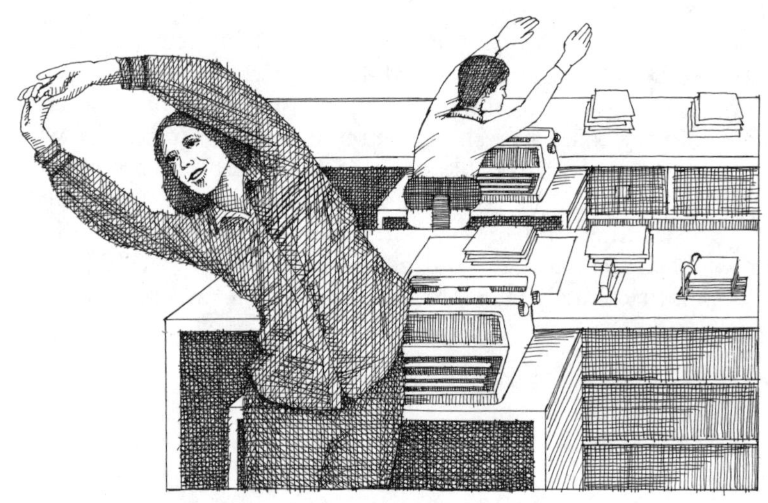

14. New Games, Dancing, Workplace Exercise

THE SO-CALLED NEW GAMES are a recent (or perhaps very old, depending upon your historical perspective) class of physical activities. They spring from the idea that sports should be playful and noncompetitive. They employ little equipment, relying instead upon the training and knowledge of leaders. Because the New Games are economical and can involve large numbers of people, many institutions, particularly schools, are finding them an attractive alternative to existing organized sports.

The noncompetitive nature of the New Games makes them look different from almost anything that we have been used to seeing on our playing fields. First, there are not likely to be spectators—only participants. Second, since the games do not require a set number of people on a team, a few or many can participate. Finally, there is a spirit of cooperation and creativity—sometimes the rules are changed in the middle of a game—and a tendency to avoid hard physical contact: "Play Hard, Play Fair, Nobody Hurt" is the New Games motto.

Probably nothing is more characteristic of the New Games than the various Earthball activities. The Earthball is a huge canvas ball filled with air. The Tournament Earthball game calls for the ball to be pushed or otherwise propelled over a goal line. When a lot of people play together, the ball is in the air most of the time. Rules may require that all participants play on their hands and knees, or that the ball be propelled only by hitting it with your buttocks ("the bump"). In a good many of the New Games, the participants are reduced to helpless laughter for a large part of the playing time, thus achieving one of the goals of the New Games movement—playfulness of the most childlike and enjoyable kind.

It's too early to tell whether the New Games are the wave of the future or just another interesting but brief event in the history of sport. Several factors make it likely that they are here to stay. For instance, there is a great need to find cheaper alternatives to the existing team sports. Outfitting a hockey or football team and providing transportation to and from games for the team, band, assorted coaches and managers, for example, soaks up a lot of community or college money.

Then there is the question of participation. Those same team sports might involve 10 to 15 percent of a school population while many of the others serve as spectators. The New Games have the advantage that everyone can participate and benefit from the physical activities. If through the Games we can teach an attitude of joyful participation at an early age and promote its continuation into adult life, the Games will have made a strong contribution to our culture.

As Dutch philosopher Johan Huizinga pointed out, play always has a tendency to be beautiful, to have rhythm and harmony. It also demands *order*—rules must be made, and deviation from them spoils the game. Because of these characteristics, play belongs to a large extent within the field of aesthetics: the same terms used to describe art can be employed to describe play—tension, poise, balance, contrast, variation, solution, and resolution. The New Games fit these criteria. But in general they are energetic forms of movement that can add much to a conditioning program. Games like Rattlers, Go-Tag, New Frisbee, or Flying Dutchman may soon become part of the American fitness repertoire.

The New Games are so varied that no particular conditioning program can be suggested. Similarly, there is little or no experience thus far with injuries, though it can be assumed that the New Games will have a low rate.

Another way of exercising with grace, form, and rhythm is dance. Dancing isn't always thought of as exercise, but it surely is, and one performance of a Polish, Ukrainian, English Morris, or other national dance group will prove to you that its members use up a lot of calories in a short time. American folk dancing, square or otherwise, ballroom dancing, ballet, disco, jazz, rock, and other types of dance are all highly energetic activities. People who participate in them regularly are often in excellent shape from a cardiovascular and muscular point of view, and their movements require a lot of flexibility as well. Dance is, in fact, one of the most potent all-around conditioning methods. A sensible way to begin, of course, is to join a group or get instruction from a qualified teacher. While we seldom think about it, ballet dancers are among the most highly developed athletes in the world. The American male bias against ballet dancing would probably change if it were identified as a male sport—but that seems a long way off.

Rhythm and melody are the motivating forces in one important exercise method, the origins of which are to be found in the Swedish Exercise Break, a ten- or fifteen-minute activity period found in most offices, factories, and other workplaces in that country. A volunteer leader brings out a tape cassette, those who wish take off their shoes if in an office or get up from the bench if in a factory, and everyone goes through a set of exercises set to music. The general effect is exhilarating, though hardly aerobic enough to work up a sweat (thus the lack of need for showers). There is a fair amount of stretching involved, and the activity is social and friendly. You don't have to participate if you don't want to, and if you think you're entitled to pastry and coffee, you can have that instead. It's just that there is a choice, and one of the choices is exercise. In Sweden, where this break is available, about 75 to 80 percent of both sexes participate. Out of this simple beginning has grown, in Scandinavia, a whole complex of workplace fitness programs, so most people have access to facilities at work as well as company encouragement to participate at their own levels.

Exercise breaks of different kinds exist in many countries, some more regimented than others (though we seem to be in the rear guard of these activities). The popular image held by Americans that all the Chinese, Japanese, and Russians are forced into a mindless daily exercise routine appears to be absolutely false; participation in most instances is voluntary.

Finally, the simplest, least expensive aerobic activity with the highest yield per minute is jumping rope. It needs no equipment other than the rope (ordinary sash cord will do, although there are ball-bearing-handled models on the market), and you can do it wherever you are. It is highly demanding, however (about three times as vigorous as jogging, for instance), so there is a danger of exceeding the target heart rate in a short time. Dr. Lenore Zohman, in her excellent pamphlet on exercise and the heart, *Beyond Diet*, recommends several methods to develop coordination (if you have never jumped before) and some training programs. As usual, your heart rate determines the level of exertion.

What characterizes the New Games, dance, workplace fitness, and jumping rope is the simplicity of application. They all provide accessible alternatives to the other fitness activities and sports we earlier described. You may find these attractive and fun, particularly for an occasional change of pace.

One of the most important goals in any fitness program is a feeling of enjoyment. Unfortunately, some programs now being developed, while based on extremely good physiology, fail to take into account the aesthetic, social, and emotional needs of potential users. The result, of course, is a high drop-out rate. Often, the only people left after an initial period of enthusiastic use are those super-fitness types who would exercise anywhere, any time, and at any price. It is not necessary to build programs for them. But there is a large, modestly motivated group of people who, with the right kind of encouragement and leadership, would join and stay in a program. Furthermore, if these programs are eclectic—changing focus now and then, providing new stimuli—they will have a better chance of success over the long run. Such alternatives should be a part of every exercise repertoire, whether or not everyone decides to use them.

III
FITNESS FOR EVERYONE

There is a danger that by emphasizing running above all other activities the public's interest and enthusiasm will wear out in a short time. After all, running isn't for everyone, and even if it were, there are sufficient reasons—wretched weather conditions in some parts of the country, for instance—that can make running a form of pure torture. There is an off-putting grimness and single-minded devotion required of certain sports that can only discourage and deter novices, even those with a well-developed sense of humor. If there is any truth in the assertion that hard-driving, ambitious people—the Type A personality—are more subject to heart attacks than relaxed, easygoing Type B folks, then it may be that running has become a haven for a lot of the A types, who simply transfer their personality characteristics to their sport, thereby offsetting any cardiovascular advantages it might otherwise offer.

The hallmark of a successful approach, whether on a national, community, or personal scale, is that it be eclectic *and* flexible, *that is, that the program allow for varying levels of participation and modes of activity. It is important that the individual participate because he/she wants to and that enough stimulation be present to maintain interest. This may mean swimming one day is the activity of choice, while tennis comes another day, followed by running. The criteria will have been met if your activity is vigorous enough to raise your pulse to levels consistent with your age and condition.*

15. Changing Our Sedentary Life-Style

ALMOST EVERYONE would agree that if the American way of life is to change from sedentary to active and health habits are to improve, these changes must originate in childhood.

The important study of Nedra Belloc and Lester Breslow, who followed over 4000 residents of Southern California for an extended period, showed that those who ate regular meals, got adequate sleep, did not drink to excess, exercised, and didn't smoke were far more likely to live longer than those who did the opposite. They not only lived longer; they also experienced much less illness, used hospitals far less often, and could be described as much more active and self-reliant. In other words, there is a significant economic benefit to living in a healthy way, an activity that ultimately benefits the entire community. Since everyone pays, through health insurance premiums and taxes, for the medical care of others, the impact of illness falls upon all of us. It is therefore in our ultimate self-interest to promote the healthiest kind of behavior.

Studies like that of Belloc and Breslow have been complemented by similar surveys of groups such as the Mormons and Seventh-Day Adventists, whose dietary habits and abstention from stimulants seem to be related to their longevity. Finally, there are the important observations of Dr. Alexander Leaf of the Massachusetts General Hospital. Leaf examined the characteristics of extremely aged individuals in three ethnic groups in different parts of the world attempting to find out why a large percentage survived beyond one hundred years. The major conclusions were: (1) each group revered the aged and looked on them as wise elders, repositories (in a predominantly oral culture) of their history and customs, (2) aging did not involve retirement from one's usual occupation, and (3) since their occupations all required large expenditures of energy (farming, hill-climbing, herding, hauling), exercise must be a major factor in preserving life.

Clearly the 130-year-old peasant who can work a full day and then settle down to an evening of folk dancing did not begin his/her exercise program at the age of fifty, eighty, or one hundred. It began as soon as he/she was able to participate fully in the work life of the community. The habits were inculcated by parents and community leaders.

In our country, instead of education by elders, the state assumes responsibility. Each school system devotes a certain amount of its budget to the building and maintenance of physical education facilities, but it is unlikely that these facilities and their teacher/coaches have been examined critically by the community at large for some time, if ever.

Much of our present fascination with competitive sports can be traced back only as far as the middle and latter parts of the nineteenth century. Our school sports are lineal descendants of British schoolboy sports, which, in turn, were introduced into the British public (i.e., private) schools in an attempt to bring order out of the educational chaos that existed up to the middle of that century. The emphasis upon competitive sports for schoolchildren has had a profound effect upon the American public. Team sports require the participation of a few, while many other students go without adequate coaching or facilities. More important, the kinds of skills taught in many schools are those having little or no relevance for later life. A reasonable question to ask concerning school sports is: Can the child use this skill when he/she is an adult, at forty, fifty, or seventy? Adults who have a large emotional investment in childhood team sports should reconsider the basis of their support for these programs, whether they are part of the school system or one of the many league-sponsored afterschool sports.

A balanced school sports program would include a larger share of lifetime, or "carryover," sports. Clearly many of the activities discussed in our earlier pages fit this description. But there is another kind of curriculum in addition to the activities themselves that could be of inestimable value to the growing child: an understanding of his/her body's physiology.

Health education has not been highly regarded by teachers or students. The old hygiene courses taught by the gym teacher or school nurse have, in some instances, been replaced by more sophisticated materials that can be taught by the regular classroom teacher. But little has been done to take advantage of the inborn need for activity all children seem to share. The tremendous energy of childhood (which, through physical fitness programs, many adults seem to be trying to recapture) could be linked to an intellectual understanding of the workings of the body by placing a version of the cardiac physiology laboratory in every school system.

Through the simple technique of taking their pulse rate, children have been taught to estimate their own level of fitness in primary grades. New curricula are being developed in some schools so that children can be taught the relationship between activity and food intake. Stories, mathematical problems, art, and music can be related to motion; physical education need not begin and end in the gym. At the high school level, the bicycle or treadmill ergometer can be used to teach physiology in a thoroughly personal way, helping the student to assess his/her own level of fitness while developing a better understanding of muscle physiology, the biochemistry of energy utilization, and cardiovascular function.

While a number of experimental attempts now exist in this country to try to reach children in this way, more needs to be encouraged. We may or may not come to the same realization that drove the Swedes, in the 1950s, to eliminate all competitive sports in schools, but we will certainly have to decide whether they are as important as we now seem to regard them.

One force for change are the Title IX regulations, which mandate equal access for females and males to all facilities. In school sports, the effect is often profound. It is too early to tell whether women are heading in the same direction as men—into elite competition—or whether school administrators can take this opportunity to reshape the entire physical education curriculum so that both men and women will receive motivation training for lifetime fitness.

In order to bring about the changes needed, physical education teachers will need a different background from the one they have traditionally received. There must be less emphasis on coaching, more on cardiovascular physiology and biochemistry. Since more and more adults are coming to use schools through the community school movement, it makes sense that teaching skills be available to this audience as well. Schools that train teachers may decide to train their students to enter the world of work with more than just the skills to lead childhood games.

It is obvious that the schools can be the focus of real institutional change. And it is up to parents and voters to demand innovation. Unfortunately, at the root of any change is the cold-blooded economic fact that it is probably too expensive and wasteful of our nation's health to continue on our present course of sports for only the very few and very gifted.

Community fitness development is really a question of facilities and leadership. The facilities need not be expensive, but if there are choices to be made between a hockey rink and a swimming pool, the safety and cardiovascular benefits of the pool should place it ahead of team hockey. This is not always the case now. Communities that must make decisions concerning new programs should be informed about the costs and benefits of these investments. Community enthusiasm for a sport, often promoted through boosters' clubs and other such interests, is often the only driving force in favor of development, when in fact reasoned arguments could be marshaled to underscore the health benefits, risks, and tradeoffs of any given activity.

The questions to be asked whenever a new sports program is planned are these:

1. Does the activity contribute to the health of its users and the community in some way?
2. Can the program be engaged in by most members of the community? The young and old? Both sexes? People with handicaps?
3. Is it fun?

Most citizens have never attended a local recreation commission meeting or, if they have, have not asked these questions. Nor have most recreation specialists or administrators thought of themselves as health specialists. But that in fact is what they *must* become if we are to have a system of health promotion. The business of maintaining health is not simply a concern of the medical profession, it is a community responsibility whose locus in the future is likely to reside at least in part with recreation experts. To insure the mental and physical health of the population is hardly the job of only the hospitals, but this is medicine's orientation presently—and likely to be for the foreseeable future.

The planning of fitness programs must take into account where people *are*. People sit. They sit at home, in their cars, in school, and at work. The job of the recreationists is to re-create, to give each person a sense of his/her body's fitness. This means bringing into action most of the unused and partially atrophied muscle that results from our way of life. This advanced state of disrepair has come about as a result of our firmly held belief that it is far better to allow some machine to do the work.

While the machine has liberated some people and raised the standard of living for many, it has exacted a terrible toll in terms of health, elevating heart disease, obesity, and back pain to alarming heights. Assuming that we are not going to give up all of our dependence on mechanical solutions and retreat into the pre-Industrial gloom, we must find ways to counteract the forces that now tend to disrupt our health.

The job, then, is to locate programs and facilities in the community through new and imaginative recreation planning. This is the responsibility of every citizen—to find ways to transform the present sports orientation of most schools into a participation model and to develop a new set of programs for workers that will develop their physical potential.

These are not radical ideas, at least not in the major part of the developed world. Countries with far fewer resources than the United States have created imaginative and attractive methods for accomplishing these goals. It is necessary to think of our culture in a new light: as an underdeveloped nation, underdeveloped in terms of its health, its ability to prevent disease, and in the level of physical competence its citizens have attained. Once that concept has been accepted, people will understand that a major investment in physical fitness can be productive. At this point, citizen demand and political reality could come together to provide the impetus for a sensible, goal-oriented set of programs.

What is needed most of all is a *fitness policy*. Even if some form of national health insurance becomes a reality, the continued rise in the cost of medical care—based largely upon advancing technology, costs of training, inflationary tendencies built into the hospital system, and the poor health of a population of increasingly older people—will demand that new and imaginative methods of preventing illness be developed. This is the basis of the present move to place the responsibility for prevention in the hands of each individual: to eat properly, to avoid cigarettes, to drink moderately or not at all, not to abuse substances. But that movement has little relevance in a population of people who have scant knowledge of how their bodies work or how to develop them. Besides, it conveys negative messages—don't do this, don't do that. If our experience with patients teaches us anything, it seems likely that eventually the public will tire of that kind of admonition, particularly when the alternatives are presented so enticingly. Nothing, for instance, rivals the skill of the cigarette companies in promoting their products, unless it is the methods used by some cereal manufacturers to persuade children to buy and eat products consisting mostly of sugar.

While some messages are negative, the message used to promote fitness is positive: it's fun, it feels good, it makes you feel good, it increases your strength and enjoyment of life. This is no exaggeration. Fitness doesn't need to be hyped to convince people that it is worthwhile. But lacking facilities and encouragement, a hard core of the population will never participate in such a movement.

The methods can be simple, the facilities inexpensive. But the major need is for leadership. This fact has been demonstrated in numerous studies. The dropout rate in most organized fitness activities is high, whether for beginners or for post-heart attack patients who probably know they would benefit from the program. As a country, we simply do not know how to lead people and engage their interest over a lifetime. To develop the right kind of leadership, our colleges and universities will have to turn from coaching and team sports as training methods in physical education to lifetime fitness. The curriculum must become more physiologically oriented, and graduates must learn how to protect the adult heart and muscles from deterioration. Health education, presently somewhere near the bottom of the secondary school curriculum heap in popularity, needs to be tied to the concept of the body in motion—in other words to become physiologically oriented.

Instead of creating a new group of paramedical professionals to carry out the mission, we must instead—using the Scandinavian model once more—develop volunteers at all levels who can lead. In every office or factory we need leaders who are themselves part of the system in which they work. Elementary classroom teachers should be able to teach and lead fitness programs instead of automatically turning their students over to a physical education teacher a few periods a week. At the community level, instruction in using fitness trails and other programs requiring some skill should be provided by people from the neighborhood who have the appropriate training and background. All of this will require backup, supervision, and professional consultation, some of it medical in nature. But it will be far better to place this knowledge in the hands of many than to reserve it for a few highly trained professionals.

The J. N. Morris and Ralph Paffenbarger studies are among the most important of their type. They illustrate the association between exercise and the prevention of heart disease. These investigations show that even a modest investment in leisure-time activities carried out by ordinary people has a marked protective effect upon the heart. As we mentioned earlier, Morris's studies in the early 1950s focused on London busdrivers and bus conductors; the two turned out to have differing death rates from heart disease. Morris believed he could correlate these differences with the amount of physical activity each group obtained at work—the drivers sitting all day, the conductors walking back and forth and climbing up to the second level of the London buses. His later investigation into heart diseases in British postal workers substantiated the earlier findings.

Powerful new evidence comes from the well-constructed studies of Dr. Ralph Paffenbarger, of Stanford University, who has shown that both groups he studied over many years—longshoremen and Harvard graduates—show striking differences in heart disease rates according to their amount of physical exertion. For instance, the 17,000 Harvard graduates studied exhibited a high rate of heart disease if sedentary in adult life (even if once active, as, for example, in college football) while those who remained active or began a physical activity as adults are relatively free from heart disease.

In medicine, we are taught to look for disease and to describe disease syndromes. Only now are we beginning to look for the roots of health instead of disease. What we do not know is: How great is the health potential of most people? Not everyone wants to become an Olympic athlete; the goal itself is totally self-serving and time-consuming. It seems to us, a proper goal is that of developing—within the existing framework of our society—a capacity for frequent, joyful exercise that is adequate to condition the body, particularly the cardiovascular system, without incurring the risk of injury.

A simple formula to remember comes in threes. The thirty minutes, three times a week schedule (plus sufficient walking) is something to which each individual, each employer, and all schools should attempt to devote time. It is difficult to think of a good reason why most people could not, given the right kind of incentives and facilities, participate in such a movement for the 1980s and after.

16. Age, Asthma, Diabetes—and Exercise

THE SPORTS FOR LIFE concept can be applied to both the healthy body and the one with limitations imposed by disease or age. Aging in itself is not abnormal, and there are fascinating unresolved questions that must be answered regarding the effect of exercise on the aging process. Furthermore, we do not yet know much about the potential for development of elderly people through exercise programs, since so few such programs exist. Finally, we are just beginning to understand that certain medical problems—asthma and diabetes are the examples we have chosen—need not limit those who wish to exercise—and indeed may benefit them.

Should a disabling condition become less disabling through fitness, either because of the improvement in muscular tone, cardiovascular endurance, or because of the psychological boost provided, sufficient justification for these programs would exist. These are new and relatively untested areas. All we can say is that since the human body was made for motion and inactivity is known to decrease its efficiency in many ways, it makes sense to enhance the potential for movement in all people, including the elderly and those with chronic illnesses that do not totally prevent movement from taking place.

AGE

Just as we must rethink our attitudes about women and exercise, we must revise our conception of age and exercise. The importance of work in this area can hardly be overstated. The elderly are a growing force in our culture. Not only are they increasing, partly as a result of better health care, but their proportion of the population becomes greater as the birth rate falls. They have become a potent political force, as any office-holder knows. Yet their earning power is poor and they are the sickest of all groups. They require more time, attention, and resources of the medical profession and have the greatest need for social services.

Nonetheless, little actual work has been done to show what effect, if any, exercise has in maintaining the health of older people. We might ask an even more important question: What effect does a lifetime of physical fitness have on the aging process? The Belloc-Breslow studies of a large population in Southern California showed that living a life of moderation, that is, not smoking, avoiding alcohol abuse (not necessarily eschewing it entirely though), eating regularly and prudently, getting enough sleep, and exercising regularly seemed to be related to living longer, and—more important—functioning better at an advanced age.

This finding has immense implications for the twenty million or so elderly persons, and for those to come, for if we could find a way to increase the self-reliance of people by even a few percentage points, billions of dollars would be saved. Exercise has that potential, but programs are often inadequate because of lack of expertise, fears (often irrational) that exercise might cause old people harm, and lack of financial commitments from those agencies that otherwise serve the elderly, particularly the housing and health complexes, as well as the bureaucracies directly concerned with affairs for the elderly.

For instance, it is almost never considered as part of the planning for an elderly housing project to place on site some form of physical fitness facility, while a common television room or "recreation room" for sedentary card games is often included. A modified outdoor exercise trail, aesthetically pleasing as well as productive in physiologic terms, might be highly cost effective, and a three-times-a-week swimming program for elderly people during the underused daytime hours at a local pool might yield significant benefits. Bus trips, now popular with elderly people, might include a programmed amount of walking or hiking, and organizations emphasizing the outdoors, such as conservation and outdoor-oriented agencies, might organize such trips. So much remains to be done that the list is almost endless.

Older people can benefit from a number of basic exercise programs. Walking is the first and most important of these. If there is poor muscular tone, lack of balance, and inflexible joints, a slow, progressive effort to counteract these problems or to assist the individual is necessary. Often this is best handled by a physical therapist or someone with similar training. A safe environment for walking is also necessary; many old people fear going outdoors because of an environment in which they are threatened by muggings or traffic accidents.

Flexibility exercises can be done at home, many of them while sitting in a chair. For those who can afford it, use of an exercise bicycle provides major improvement of cardiovascular endurance as well as leg muscles. If the Internal Revenue Service accepts the three-martini lunch as a deductible item for business people, then it is not too large a conceptual leap to imagine a similar deduction for people who wish to maintain their fitness by purchasing an exercise bike.

Dance—mostly square and ballroom dancing—is a natural way of enhancing the movement of old people and has valuable social functions as well. Swimming, with its relative weightlessness, is also an excellent conditioner for the elderly. In addition, it is free of some of the potential injury-producing effects of certain other sports.

Aged bones can be brittle, and joints often lack resiliency and flexibility. A fall can result in a broken hip or other major disability. These facts must be taken into consideration, while at the same time encouraging physical activity to help improve musculoskeletal tone. For many elderly people who have not exercised regularly, a careful evaluation by a trained therapist will be an important first step. After that, the success of any program will depend largely upon the skill and enthusiasm of the leader.

Chief among the remedial exercises that should be brought to bear on the elderly population immediately are joint flexibility maneuvers. The older person is often characterized by his/her lack of a full range of motion in a number of joints. Usually, this begins with a little joint inflammation, from arthritis or bursitis; soon the person has unconsciously limited his/her motion in the joint. After a surprisingly short time, the joint is "frozen"—that is, it cannot extend or rotate through its normal range of motion. It may be adequate for activities of the usual limited variety carried out by our elderly, but not for a vigorous life.

Because most elderly are inactive, their degeneration is almost guaranteed. Muscles and bones, as we have pointed out, are not static pieces of machinery; they are constantly in flux, building up or down, or being molded by physical forces about them, including gravity. Therefore, sitting in a chair or lying in bed for days at a time, or even riding in a car, enhances the degenerative process, whether for young or old. As we earlier pointed out in referring to Dr. Alexander Leaf's studies, in some cultures old people aren't forced to retire at some arbitrary age; they maintain a position of respect and prominence in their cultures or tribes. They keep active, too, by herding sheep or farming, often climbing steep mountains with the agility of young athletes, leaving less well trained observers from our industrialized society panting in the rear. Their fitness is an integral part of their health and productivity.

Even though there is a wide range of variability in aerobic capacity at various ages, certain inevitable changes take place with advanced age. Maximal muscle strength, for instance, is reached between the ages of twenty and thirty, and then begins to wane, so that the muscle strength of the average sixty-five-year-old person is about 80 percent of the peak level. Training can affect these levels, however; a Canadian fitness promotional campaign done several years ago made much of the fact that an average sixty-year-old Swede was as fit as the typical twenty-nine-year-old Canadian male.

Aerobic power decreases with age as well, but this is again subject to much individual variation related to training and natural endowment. The most critical period, as determined through the investigations of Åstrand and his co-workers, is between ten and twenty years of age. The effort spent at that time to develop aerobic power appears to be a major determinant of later capacity. Aligned with the drop of aerobic power is the decline in maximal pulse rate, which appears to be independent of training. The lowered ceiling for heart rate that occurs as one gets older may be nature's way of protecting the heart against exposure to a workload that could be inappropriate to the heart's capacity to respond. Since it has been shown that breathing pure oxygen during these exertions does not improve performance in older individuals, it must be concluded that the lower heart rate is not a consequence of *lack* of oxygen so much as it is a consequence of impaired lung function, although the lungs, too, lose some of their elasticity (and thus the capacity to transport oxygen) with age.

While aging may be associated with some inevitable changes, resulting in the lessening of physical capacities, the medical profession has applied little expertise toward the improvement of the physical status of elderly people. This is in part because the profession is oriented toward disease rather than wellness. There is, however, a movement toward the definition of health, and some practitioners are practicing what they refer to as wellness-oriented medicine. Though this number is small, it should give hope to people interested in the subject to know that there are some outstanding examples of very fit behavior among older people. With the new emphasis on community-based sports, such as running, more and more older people are turning up in races, doing well in competition, and thereby disproving the myth of deterioration. Senior Olympics programs or masters' competitions have begun to appear in a number of areas as well, giving some evidence of greater emphasis upon fitness for the elderly.

As we said, the real need is for competent research and evaluation. We need to know whether, for good and sound economic reasons, the elderly can be brought to higher levels of self-sufficiency and self-esteem by participation in regular physical activity.

ASTHMA

Asthma, a disabling lung disorder characterized by wheezing and shortness of breath, affects about four million people in the United States. Usually, its occurrence is obvious, since the breath sounds of an acute attack are unlike any other noises heard through the physician's stethoscope. What is less clear, however, is the diagnosis of exercise-induced asthma.

This type of lung disease is often quite subtle, and because it appears only on exertion, its diagnosis may be difficult. In a sedentary society, those who never exert themselves may never have symptoms of their disease. While this seems at first glance like a good thing, it has its costs.

Usually the condition appears early in life and the child soon learns that exertion causes discomfort, though the disorder is not known. He/she will find ways of avoiding exercise and is likely to become a withdrawn, solitary, unathletic person, particularly if her/his contemporaries are active themselves, as most children are. The tragedy of these children is they become fixed in an inactive way of life—knowing they can't compete, they drop out. Their physicians may be unaware of the diagnosis, and parents may attribute their behavior to a lack of competitiveness or "drive." As adults, they risk becoming fat and poorly trained from both a cardiovascular and a musculoskeletal point of view: good candidates for the diseases of disuse. They adapt to the workplace as they did to school—by avoiding movement. They believe they are ideally suited to desk jobs. Because they do not know they have asthma, they are not likely to improve. With diagnosis and treatment, their world can immediately expand. Asthma is one condition in which drug treatment can be genuinely liberating.

Fortunately, by itself asthma is no reason to avoid exercise.

Most asthmatics show no deterioration of lung function even as the result of repeated attacks. If treatment can prevent attacks during exercise, the asthmatic's capacity to exercise may be as great as any other person's. In fact, a number of asthmatics compete regularly in Olympic events, and the Olympic committee has sanctioned several antiasthma drugs that can be used by competitors.

Although drugs are important in treatment, so is training. There is considerable reason for hope that by training an asthmatic can improve her/his performance. However, free running of *over* six minutes is the most potent stimulus to the development of asthma in susceptible persons. Thus, short-duration training periods are desirable and have been shown to be effective. Lung function certainly is improved by this type of interval training. Most programs emphasize a combination of running and rest, or running and walking. The intervals should be short—two minutes of running and four minutes of walking, for instance, building up to five minutes of running with ten minutes of walking or rest. Eventually, improved tolerance for exercise results. Through such a program the asthmatic will be able to increase cardiovascular endurance considerably.

The role of drugs in treatment of exercise-induced asthma is well established. Two drugs approved by the International Olympic Committee are terbutaline and cromolyn sodium. Either of these, taken before exercise, is likely to prevent attacks of crippling asthma. Theophyllines (the most common of which is aminophylline) are also very useful if given prior to exercise.

DIABETES

It has long been recognized that exercise affects the diabetic by lowering blood sugar, but most textbook descriptions of the disease do little to foster useful activity. It is also true that an athlete can have diabetes and yet succeed in sports. What is required is a close working knowledge of the disorder, combined with some skill and flexibility in handling diet, medications, and exercise to avoid the complications of overdose and poor diabetic control.

The stable diabetic is likely to be middle-aged or older, and approximately 95 percent of such diabetics are obese. Weight reduction is very important. Fortunately, a large number of these people can control their diabetes with diet alone, and in some cases evidence of the disease disappears with weight reduction and proper diet. We have already talked about the important role exercise plays in burning calories. It should be obvious that for the obese diabetic, exercise is essential as part of the comprehensive approach to better health—supplementing the meal plan.

The unstable diabetic presents more challenges. While we cannot here provide a handbook on the treatment of unstable diabetes, it should be said that exercise has a role in the life of this type of diabetic, particularly if certain cautions are observed.

If insulin is injected into a part of the body used for vigorous movement, such as the leg, absorption into the system may be speeded up to a dangerous level by exercise. A sudden burst of insulin, occurring particularly at the time of exercise, which itself (if sustained) can lower blood sugar, may cause insulin reaction. For this reason, it is better to inject the hormone into the abdominal wall, or the fatty area of the buttock.

Most specialists in diabetes who treat athletes will allow the athlete to run a slightly high blood sugar level just before exercise. The unstable diabetic is encouraged to eat before exercise and to have a glucose supplement hourly during prolonged exercise. After some experience, diabetic exercisers will adjust their diabetes during exercise by eating more rather than by dropping their dose of insulin.

However, when beginning a regular exercise program, diabetics should reduce their insulin dose by about 20 to 40 percent, then test their urine four times a day to establish control. One major precaution is that if evidence of acidosis exists (the presence of ketones in the urine is suggestive here), the normal mechanisms of control may be working improperly and exercise will aggravate the diabetic condition. This can lead to ketoacidosis and diabetic coma. On the other hand, if there is too much insulin, energy supply to the muscles may be impaired.

All this is to say that diabetes, even the unstable variety, is no bar to exercise. But the athletic diabetic patient should be cared for by someone who is knowledgeable in both diabetic treatment and the effect of physical activity upon the diabetic.

Appendix

WHAT TO EXERCISE

Strengthening

	Neck	Shoulder	Upper Arm	Lower Arm	Back	Abdomen	Groin	Hip	Quadriceps	Hamstrings	Calf	Foot
Walking, Running						●		●	●	●		●
Racquet Sports		●	●	●	●	●	●	●	●	●	●	●
Swimming		●	●	●	●			●				
Downhill Skiing					●	●		●	●	●		●
Cross-Country Skiing		●	●	●	●	●		●	●	●	●	●
Bicycling	●	●			●	●		●	●	●	●	
Canoeing, Kayaking		●	●		●							
Rowing		●	●		●				●	●	●	●
Football	●	●	●	●	●	●	●	●	●	●	●	
Rugby	●	●	●	●	●	●	●	●	●	●	●	
Soccer	●				●	●	●	●	●	●	●	●
Basketball					●	●	●	●	●	●	●	●
Baseball		●	●	●	●	●	●	●	●	●	●	●
Ice Sports			●	●	●		●	●	●	●	●	●

Stretching

	Neck	Shoulder	Low Back, Trunk	Groin	Quadriceps	Hamstrings	Calf
Walking, Running			•			•	•
Racquet Sports		•	•	•	•	•	•
Swimming	•	•	•	•			
Downhill Skiing		•	•	•		•	•
Cross-Country Skiing		•	•	•	•	•	•
Bicycling	•	•	•		•	•	•
Canoeing, Rowing		•	•		•		
Football	•	•	•	•	•	•	•
Rugby	•	•	•	•	•	•	•
Soccer	•		•	•	•	•	•
Basketball			•	•	•	•	•
Baseball		•	•	•	•	•	•
Ice Sports			•	•	•		•

HOW TO EXERCISE

Strengthening

Strengthening exercises should be done 3 to 4 times per week.

NECK

Neck strengthening should be done in 6 directions: bending forward and back, tilting to each side, and rotating in each direction. In each exercise, resistance to the movement is provided by the athlete's or a partner's hands in such a fashion that the head slowly moves through the complete arc of motion over an 8- to 10-second interval. This is a combined isometric and dynamic exercise. As the neck muscles get stronger, increased resistance to movement is applied even though the duration of the exercise remains the same.

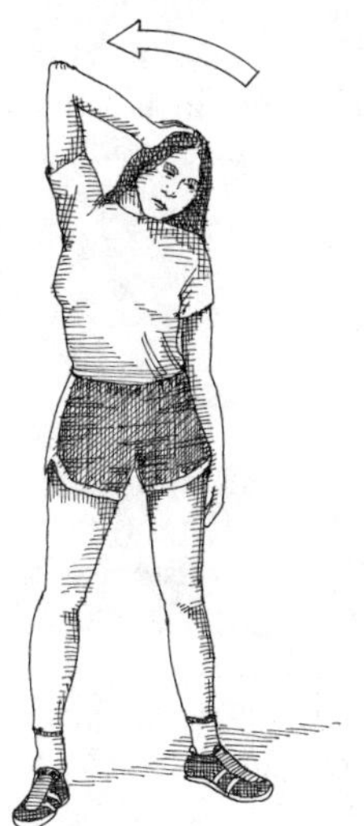

Neck strengthening using
the right hand for resistance

SHOULDERS

Since the shoulder is a nearly "universal" joint, with arcs of motion in the horizontal and vertical planes of 270 degrees, strengthening must be done

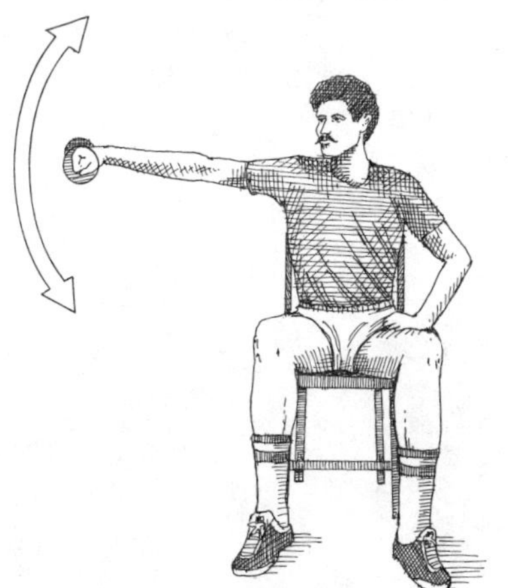

Shoulder strengthening using
a hand dumbbell

in the arcs of motion required by one's sport. Hand dumbbells, wall pulleys, chest springs, or exercise machines can all be used to attain progressive strengthening. The arm is held in the fully straightened position. The athlete may be standing, sitting, or lying down while performing the exercise. Do 3 sets of 7 to 10 repetitions.

UPPER ARMS

a. The muscles in the front of the arm that flex the elbow are strengthened by bending the arm from the fully straightened to the fully bent position, against resistance. Resistance can be provided by single hand dumbbells, two handed barbells, springs, or wall pulleys. To do an arm curl, the arm is slowly moved into the fully flexed position over a 3-second count, and slowly extended over a 5-second count, using the amount of weight or resistance that can be lifted for 7 to 10 repetitions of the exercise. Once again, these can be performed while standing, sitting, or lying on the back.

b. The muscles that extend or straighten the elbow are strengthened in exactly the opposite fashion from those in front. The elbow is straightened against progressively increasing resistance over a 3-second count and lowered over a 5-second count. Do 7 to 10 repetitions. The bench press and the sitting press are examples of this type of exercise. In the sitting press, the weights are lowered behind the head to the shoulder, for maximum benefit.

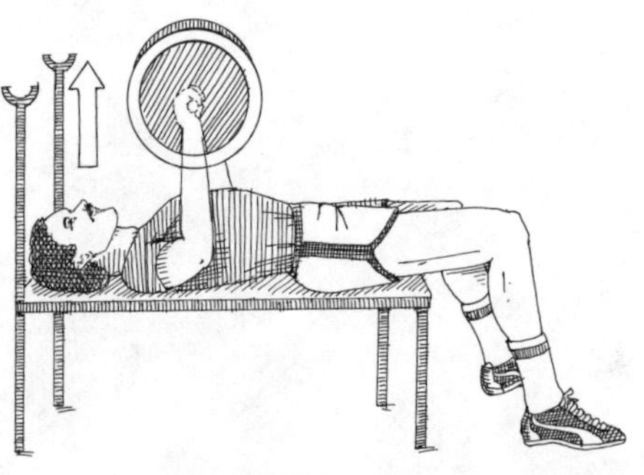

Bench press

LOWER ARM, OR FOREARM

a. The muscles of the front and back of the forearm are responsible for flexing and extending the wrists and fingers, respectively. Those in front are strengthened by bending the wrist up against resistance, while the extensor muscles in back are strengthened by wrist extension. Do 3 sets of 7 to 10 repetitions.

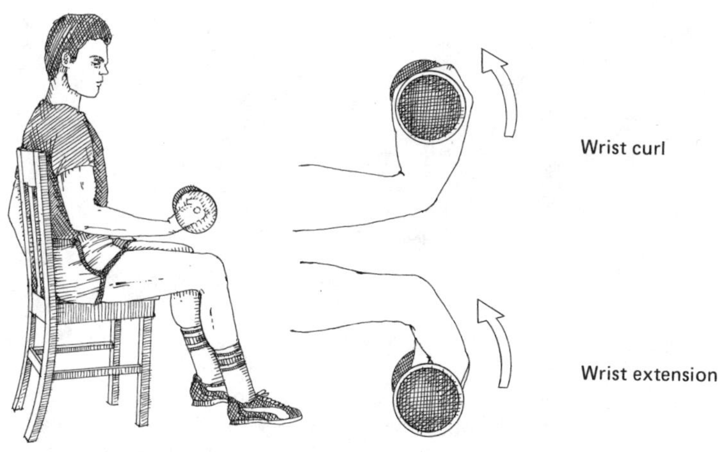

b. Hand strengthening: The small muscles of the hand and the forearm muscles controlling the hand can be simultaneously strengthened by repetitive squeezing of a rubber ball, tennis ball, heavy playdough, or "Silliputty." Do 3 sets of 10 repetitions with each hand, alternating hands.

BACK

a. The pelvic tilt is the foundation of all back strengthening and flexibility programs. Lie on back with knees and hips bent. Flatten back against floor. Hold for 10 seconds. Do 10 times.

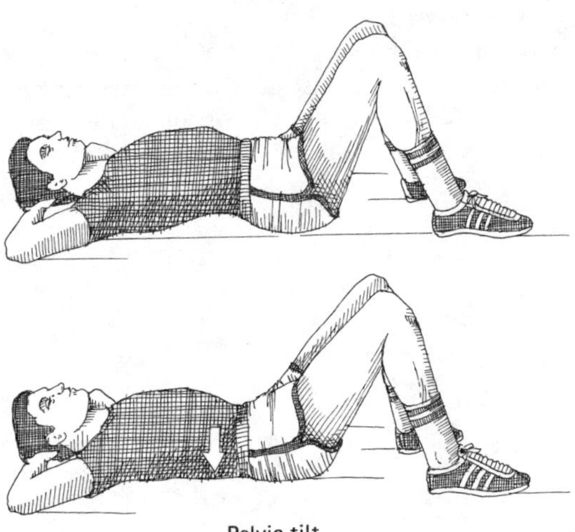

Pelvic tilt

This can also be done standing anywhere. At first, practice against a wall.

b. Back extensions (the "fish"): Lie on stomach with hands behind head. Lift elbows, squeeze shoulder blades together, and elevate chest from floor. Hold for 10 seconds at first, increasing finally to 30 seconds. Do 5 to 10 times.

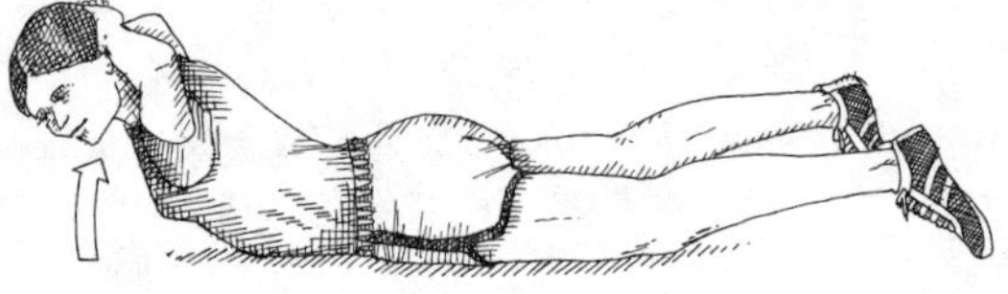

The "fish"

This can also be done from the standing position. Grasp hands behind back, bend forward at the waist, and then straighten. This can be performed as a progressive resistance exercise by supporting weights behind the head and extending against their resistance. Do 7 to 10 times. Progressively increase the weight as strength increases.

ABDOMINALS

a. The sit-up is the primary abdominal strengthening exercise. Lie on your back with the hips and knees bent. Slowly roll up to a sit-up. At first, only clear shoulder blades. As strength increases, proceed to a full sit-up. Always do slowly, without jerking or arching of the back. Do as many as you can do smoothly, increasing repetitions up to a maximum of 50 as strength increases.

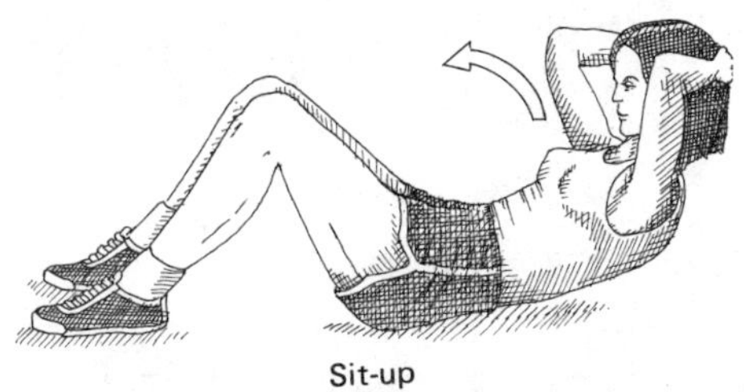

Sit-up

b. Bicycle: Lie on your back with knees bent. Lift legs and bicycle. At first, do for 10 to 15 seconds. Increase to 3 minutes as strength increases. Always keep back flattened (pelvic tilt).

c. Leg Lifts: Lie on your back with one leg bent and one straight. Slowly lift straight leg to a right angle. Keep back flat. Do 3 sets of 10 repetitions with each leg, alternating legs.

GROIN

The groin muscles are on the inside of each leg and move the hips inward.

a. Sit on the floor with knees bent and the soles of your feet together. Spread legs apart as far as possible, bend forward, and place each bent elbow against the inside of its knee. Slowly move knees together while resisting with elbows. Do 3 sets of 10 repetitions, each repetition lasting 10 seconds in duration.

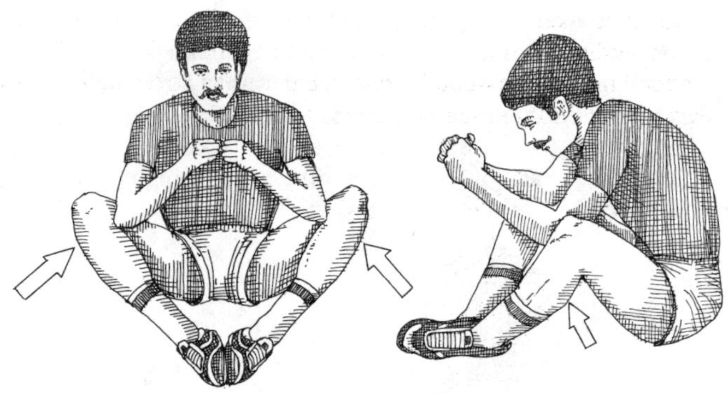

Groin strengthening

b. Lie on back with arms spread and palms down. Raise your legs up to a right angle, slowly spread them apart as far as possible, then bring them together. Do 3 sets of 7 to 10 repetitions.

HIPS

a. Hip flexors: The straight leg raising exercise described for the back and trunk also strengthens the flexor muscles of the hip. In addition, the standing marching exercise, in which each leg is raised as high as possible while slowly marching in place, should be done. Do for 1 minute initially, increasing by 15-second intervals up to a maximum of 5 minutes as strength increases.

b. Hip extenders—the squat: Do half knee bends, bending at the knees while keeping the back straight until the thighs are parallel to the ground, then slowly stand upright. Do 8 to 10 repetitions, initially, and add repetitions as strength increases. Or, do as a progressive resistance exercise by performing with barbell and weights held across the shoulder, performing 7 to 10 repetitions, and adding weight to the barbells as strength increases.

QUADRICEPS

The quadriceps muscle in the front of the thigh straightens the knee. Both the straight leg raising and squat exercises help strengthen the quads. In addition, dynamic knee extensions can be done while sitting on a high chair or table and raising the leg to full extension. This is done as a progressive resistance exercise by hanging an old handbag or paint can from the foot and adding as much weight as can be lifted. Do 7 to 10 times. Weight is added in 1- to 2-pound increments per week as strength increases. Total weight should not exceed 30 pounds for each leg.

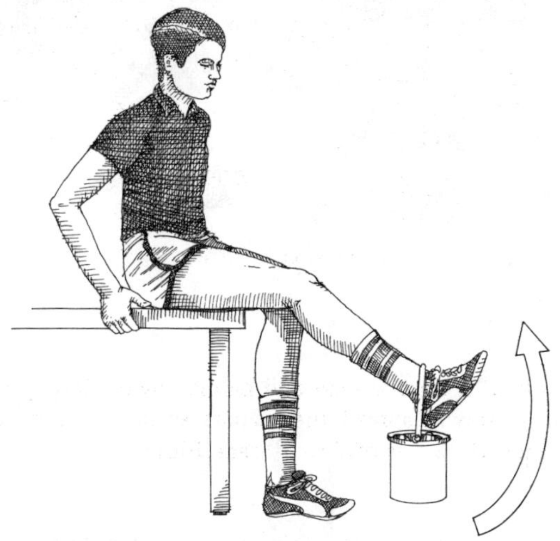

Dynamic knee extension

THE HAMSTRINGS

The hamstring muscles flex the knee. They are strengthened by performing leg curls using free weights or by the exercise machines for progressive resistance. Lie flat on the abdomen with the legs straight. Slowly bend the legs as far as possible. Do 7 to 10 times, increasing resistance as strength increases. An exercise weight boot can be used for convenience.

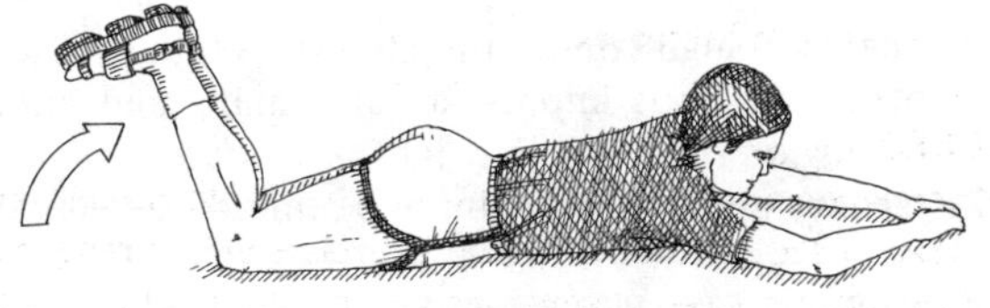

Leg curls using an exercise weight boot for resistance

CALF MUSCLES

a. Back of the calf: The powerful gastrocnemius and soleus muscles are connected to the heel by the Achilles' tendon. They are strengthened by toe raises in which the athlete slowly rises up onto the toes over a 3-second count and then returns to the flat foot position over a 5-second count. This exercise can be made more effective by placing a

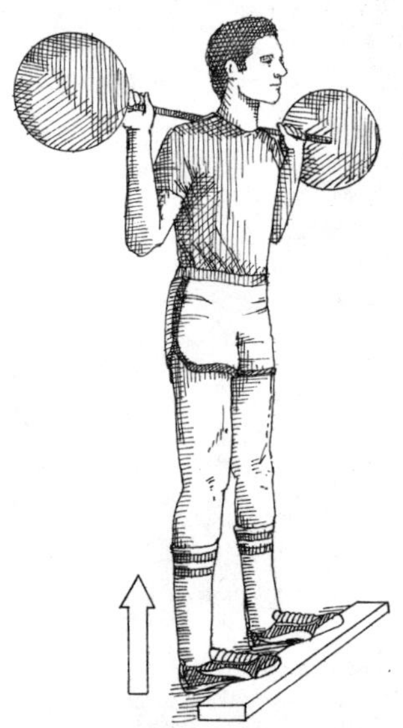

Toe raise onto a 2 x 4
using a barbell for resistance

length of 2 by 4 under the toes and rising up onto this. This should be done 20 times initially, adding repetitions up to a maximum of 50 as strength increases, or done as a progressive resistance exercise by supporting a barbell and weights on the shoulders, performing 7 to 10 repetitions, and adding weights progressively as strength increases.

b. Front of the calf: Maintaining the strength of the muscles that flex up the foot and ankle is important for running and jumping. This is done by walking on the heels, initially for 30 seconds, and then increasing by 15 seconds up to a maximum of 5 minutes as strength increases.

FOOT MUSCLES

a. A simple exercise for strengthening the muscles of the foot is picking up pebbles or marbles with the toes for 1 to 2 minutes.

b. Another series of exercises for the foot muscles can be performed sitting down. Get a 2' loop of ½" rubber tubing, tie it to itself, and place it over the front of each foot. Pivoting on your heels, slowly roll out each foot over a 3-second count, then roll each foot in over a 5-second count, using the opposite foot as resistance. The muscles on the inside of the foot and ankle can be strengthened by lifting the legs a foot off the ground, crossing them, placing the tubing over the feet, and again rolling the feet in and out. Do 3 sets of 10 repetitions.

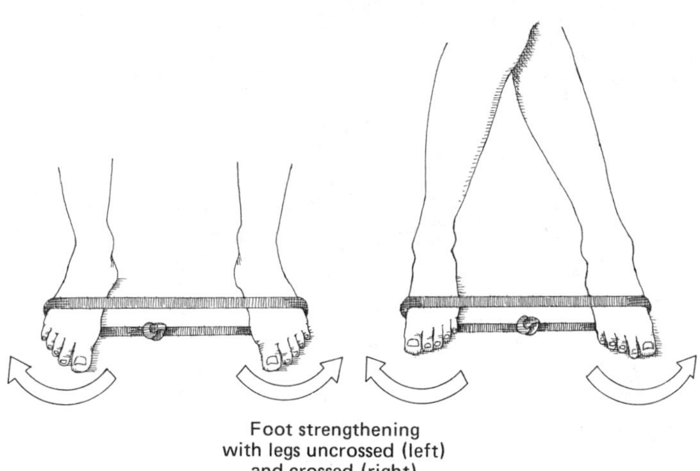

Foot strengthening with legs uncrossed (left) and crossed (right)

Stretching

Stretching exercises should be done once or twice a day, 7 days a week.

NECK

Flexibility of the neck is maintained by slow ranging of the neck in its six motions of flexion, extension, downward tilting to the left and right, and rotations in both directions. This is done over 10 to 15 seconds in each direction, and only the muscles of the neck are used to do the ranging.

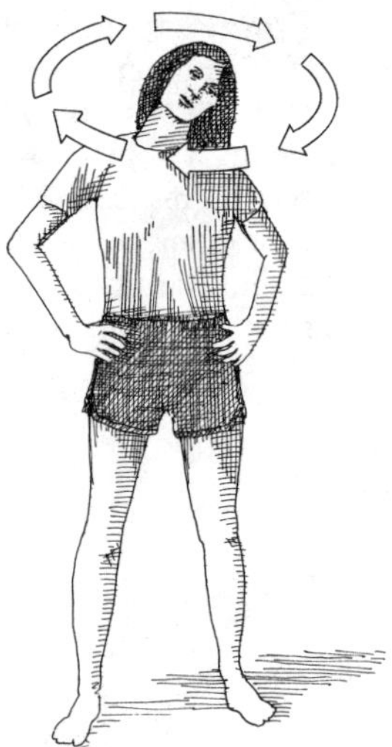

Neck ranging

SHOULDERS

a. One of the simplest shoulder stretching exercises is hanging from a bar, with all muscles relaxed, for 8 to 10 seconds.

b. The second recommended technique is done with the help of a broomstick. Grasping the stick horizontally in front with hands apart and palms down, the stick is slowly elevated as far as possible over 10 to 12 seconds and then lowered over the same count. It is then rotated in both directions. These maneuvers are repeated with palms up. Finally, the stick is placed behind the back, raised as far as possible, rotated, and lowered. Do 3 sets.

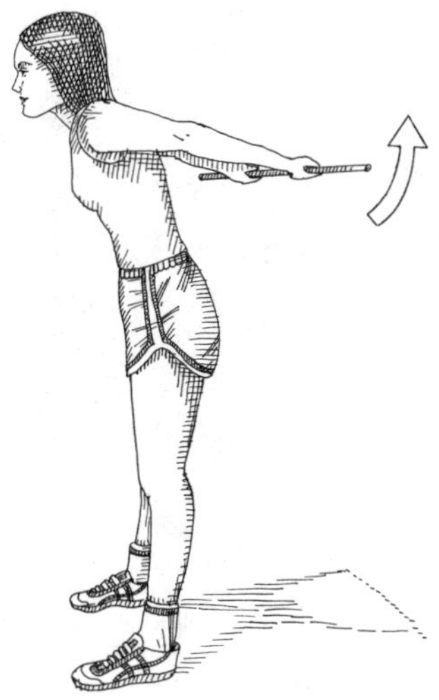

Shoulder stretch
with a broomstick behind
the back

LOW BACK AND TRUNK

These stretches can be done both lying down or standing up.

a. The simplest low back stretch is the knee-chest stretch, in which you lie on your back, draw the knees up slowly, and grasp them with the arm. The legs are then slowly straightened and lowered to the floor one at a time over a 10-second count, while the other leg remains flexed to stretch the front of each hip. Do 3 to 5 repetitions with each leg.

b. Standing stretches of the low back and trunk begin by slowly bending forward from the waist with your hands behind your back to concentrate the stretch on the low back. Maintain this position for 10 to 15 seconds. Repeat the stretch to the bent position and slowly laterally bend and rotate the spine in each direction. Finally, the exercise is completed by arching the back posteriorly. Repeat the entire sequence 3 times. This exercise is also good for stretching the hamstrings.

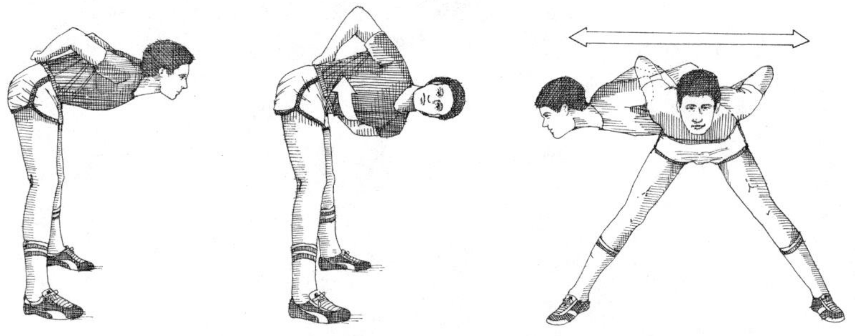

Standing low back and trunk stretch
forward stretch (left)
rotated stretch (center)
lateral stretch (right)

GROIN

Groin stretches are done both standing and sitting.

a. While standing, spread the legs as widely as possible and then bend forward from the waist, first extending the trunk down over one leg and then over the other, maintaining each position for 8 to 10 seconds. Repeat 3 to 5 times.

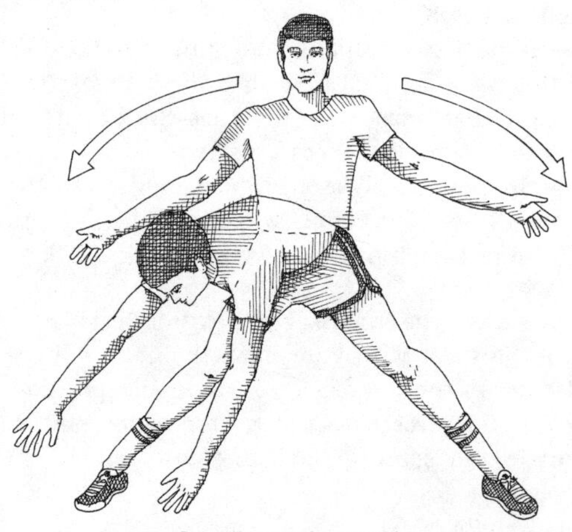

Standing groin stretch

b. From the sitting position, with the back straight, bend up the legs and place the soles of the feet against each other. Slowly draw the feet in toward the buttocks, and, while doing so, place each elbow against its own knee and push the knees toward the floor, maintaining an 8- to 10-second slow stretch. Repeat 3 to 5 times.

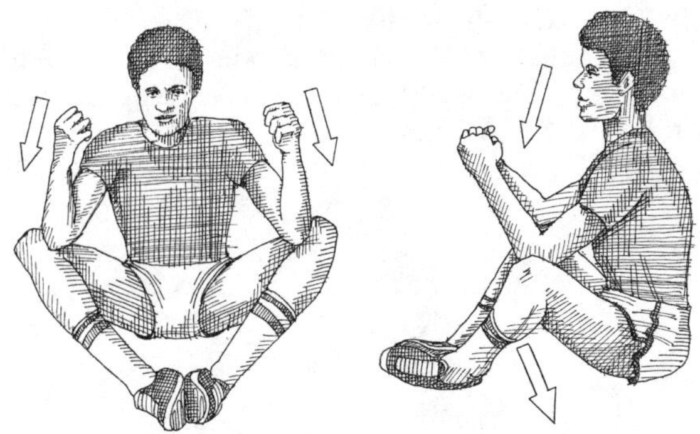

Sitting groin stretch

QUADRICEPS

Can be done either lying face down or standing.

a. When stretching lying down, lie face down on a firm surface, flex up both knees, grasp both ankles, and pull gently for 8 to 10 seconds. Maintain the chest and chin on the floor to prevent arching of the back. Repeat 3 to 5 times.

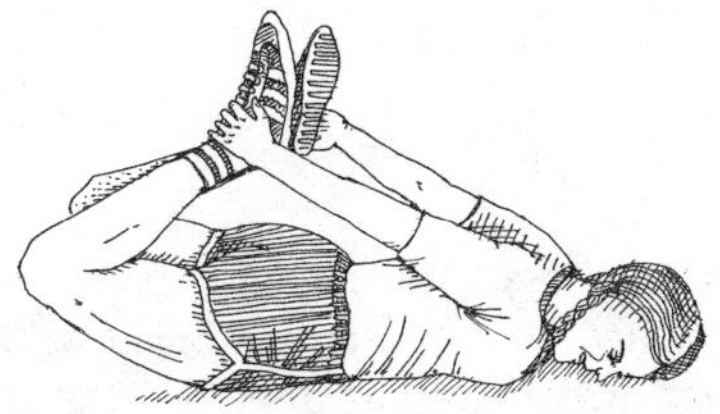

Quadriceps stretch lying down

b. To stretch standing up, stand on one leg, flex up the opposite knee with the foot behind the back, grasp the ankle with the same hand,

and slowly draw up the ankle and foot to the back of the leg. Maintain the stretch for 8 to 10 seconds. Alternate legs. Repeat 3 to 5 times.

HAMSTRINGS (back of the thigh)

a. Sit with feet out in front and legs extended, grasp the hands behind the back, and slowly bend forward while keeping the shoulder blades together. Repeat 3 to 5 times.

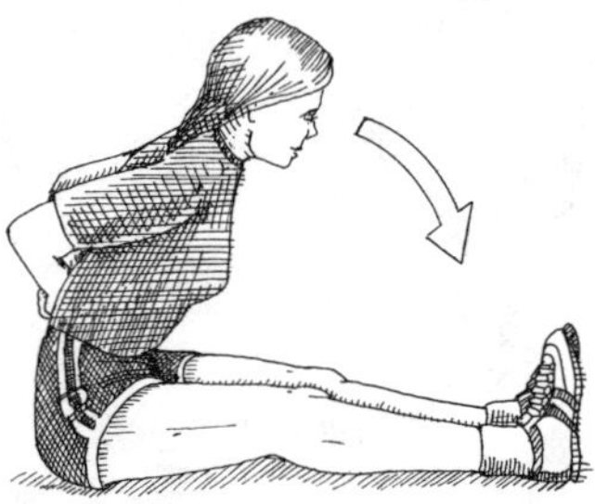

Hamstrings stretch

b. Stand opposite a table or fence at waist level, rest the ankle of one straight leg on the table, and slowly bend forward from the waist over the extended leg for 8 to 10 seconds. Alternate legs. Repeat 3 to 5 times.

CALF

Stand squarely facing a wall, fence, or partner, position each foot 18 inches apart and turned in 15 degrees. Begin at 4 feet from the wall. Slowly lean forward while keeping the heels against the floor and the knees, hips, and back straight. Maintain the maximum forward lean possible for 8 to 10 seconds. Repeat 3 to 5 times. The distance from the wall may be increased as the calves become more flexible.

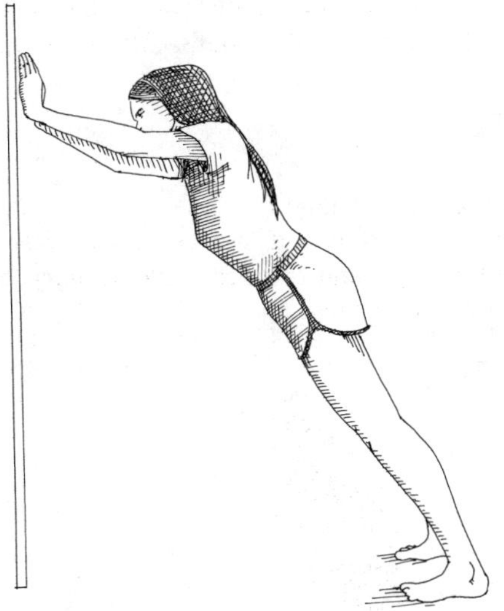

Calf stretch

For Further Information

American White Water Safety Code. American White Water, P.O. Box 1584, San Bruno, California 94066.

Amsterdam, E. A., Wilmore, J. H., and DeMaria, A. N., eds. *Exercise in Cardiovascular Health and Disease.* New York: Yorke Medical Books, 1977.

Åstrand, Per-Olof, M.D., *Health and Fitness.* Woodbury, NY, Barron's, 1977.

Åstrand, Per-Olof, M.D., and Rodahl, K. *Textbook of Work Physiology: Physiological Bases of Exercise.* New York: McGraw-Hill, 1977.

Caldwell, John, *Caldwell on Cross Country.* Brattleboro, VT: Stephen Greene Press, 1976.

Cooper, Kenneth H., M.D., M.P.H. *The New Aerobics.* New York: Bantam, 1970.

Fluegelman, A., ed. *The New Games Book.* Garden City, NY: Dolphin Books/Doubleday, 1976.

Hines, Henry. *Quick Tennis.* New York: Dutton, 1977.

Katch, F. I., and McArdle, W. D. *Nutrition, Weight Control, and Exercise.* Boston: Houghton Mifflin, 1977.

Norman, Dean, ed. *The All Purpose Guide to Paddling.* Matteson, IL: Great Lakes Living Press, 1976.

Peterson, James A., ed. *Conditioning for a Purpose.* West Point, NY: Leisure Press, 1977.

Shepro, David, and Knuttgen, Howard. *Complete Conditioning: The No-Nonsense Guide to Fitness and Good Health.* Reading, MA: Addison-Wesley, 1976.

Smith, N. J. *Food for Sport.* Palo Alto, CA: Bull Publishing Company, 1976.

Wilkerson, J. A., ed. *Medicine for Mountaineering.* The Mountaineers, 719 Pike Street, Seattle, WA 1978.

Zohman, Lenore R., M.D. *Beyond Diet: Exercise Your Way to Fitness and Heart Health.* CPC International, Inc., 1974. Single copies available from your American Heart Association.

Index